Making it in British Medicine

Essential guidance for international doctors

A06581

Sabina Dosani

MBBS MSc MRCPsych
Specialist Registrar in Child and Adolescent Psychiatry
Maudsley Hospital, London

and

Peter Cross

Writer and Journalist

Foreword by
Sir Graeme Catto
President
General Medical Council

Radcliffe Publishing
Oxford • San Francisco

Radcliffe Publishing Ltd
18 Marcham Road
Abingdon
Oxon OX14 1AA
United Kingdom

www.radcliffe-oxford.com
Electronic catalogue and worldwide online ordering facility.

British Library Cataloguing in Publication Data

A catalogue record for this book is available from the British Library.

ISBN 1 85775 875 7

Typeset by Advance Typesetting Ltd, Oxfordshire
Printed and bound by TJ International Ltd, Padstow, Cornwall

Contents

Foreword

For many years the United Kingdom, and the NHS in particular, has depended on International doctors to help keep the nation healthy.

It is not uncommon to find doctors from four continents working within the same medical firm. Migration to a new country and a new culture is never going to be without its problems and anything that attempts to make things easier is to be welcomed.

Although the principal role of the GMC in relation to doctors entering the medical profession is to set standards and assess competencies, we recognise that there needs to be significant improvements to the information and guidance that is provided for International medical graduates contemplating coming to the UK.

As part of our contribution to bringing this about we have been asking successful PLAB candidates a year after passing the test to let us have their views about their experience in gaining their first and subsequent posts. The results of these surveys will be used to inform the material we provide for future PLAB candidates.

We are keen to work with others better placed than ourselves to ensure that doctors contemplating a move to the UK have adequate information about training and employment opportunities on which to base their decision. This can just as readily be organisations like the Department of Health and NHS Professionals as it can individuals with first-hand experience of what it takes to secure their first SHO post.

This book specifically sets out to help International doctors consider options available here, both to train and to practise, within the British healthcare system. This practical guide is full of helpful information and good advice; the sort of help that might make the difference between a positive and negative experience.

While the UK welcomes doctors and other professionals trained abroad wishing to work here, the requirements and eccentricities of British life can seem confusing and very different from what they know from home. But many International doctors have made fulfilling careers for themselves in the NHS and have found the UK a good place to live and work.

Sir Graeme Catto
President
General Medical Council
August 2004

Preface

Go confidently in the direction of your dreams. Live the life you have imagined.

Henry David Thoreau (1817–1862)

It is not often that you can recall the exact moment when an idea was conceived. But this book's conception can be pinpointed to the 2002 *British Medical Journal* (*BMJ*) Careers Fair in London.

Sabina was helping on the *BMJ* Careers stall and spent much of her time fielding numerous questions from a procession of foreign doctors. These doctors, who were in various states of agitation and bewilderment, were desperate for information about the British medical system as they attempted to establish a career in the United Kingdom (UK). Many were baffled by what they had discovered and their dream of starting a new life was turning into a nightmare. Much of the agitation was due to having invested considerable time, effort and money in coming to Britain yet not being able to find the quality training and employment they sought.

Many of these doctors didn't understand the different roles played by the General Medical Council (GMC), Royal Colleges and British Medical Association (BMA), and were understandably confused.

Seeing Britain and British institutions through foreign eyes is illuminating. People who have lived in Britain for all or most of their lives are used to the quirky and confusing ways, think little of it, and indeed find it difficult to imagine life differently. This book has been written to provide answers to some of the questions put to Sabina and, perhaps more importantly, to put those answers in a context that will make British medicine and British life more understandable.

Our research has been a journey of discovery for us as well. We knew nothing of the International English Language Testing System (IELTS) or the Professional Linguistic Assessment Board (PLAB) at the onset. We only had a cursory knowledge about the different Royal Colleges, their membership exams and differences between them.

Official guidance is frequently difficult to understand. Where necessary we have converted this information into flow charts. We have interviewed over a hundred people for this book and their helpful contributions pepper the text and certainly helped us make sense of how you unravel British red tape to achieve a worthwhile career or training.

We have concentrated on the National Health Service (NHS) as most health jobs and almost all appropriate training take place in this huge organisation. There is some private health provision in the UK and you also find private employers with NHS contracts, but most doctors working in Britain come under the NHS umbrella one way or another. While we describe the NHS in Chapter 2 as a lumbering giant staggering from crisis to crisis, we both feel that there is something very commendable about it, making it an organisation worth working and fighting for.

While writing this book, Sabina was involved in a piece of research for the *BMJ*, investigating advertisements for so-called 'trust grade' doctors. In essence these are unrecognised posts that various NHS trusts have created and are using to fill the growing gap that exists between medical needs and service availability of doctors in training. It soon became clear that the group being targeted qualified outside the UK. We hope that this book will alert international and overseas doctors to the shortcomings of these jobs.

It is worth mentioning here how we define overseas and international doctors. An overseas doctor is one who does not have settled status or a right of indefinite residence in the UK. European Economic Area (EEA) nationals who have gained their primary medical qualifications in an EEA member state are not overseas doctors by this definition. We have used the term 'international doctors' to refer to both overseas doctors and EEA nationals. Conversely, when rules or regulations apply only to overseas doctors, we refer to them specifically. The GMC, however, tend to refer to 'International medical graduates' as doctors who do not benefit from European law.

Medicine is still one of the most prestigious professions in Britain. Despite increasing competition from an ever-expanding legal profession, information technology (IT) industry and other dynamic young industries and the media, medical schools are still able to select the cream of the nation's youth. If this is true, it follows that it will be additionally difficult for someone who has graduated abroad. British-trained doctors have home advantage, know the culture and speak English fluently. Some specialties are much more competitive than others.

But the climate is fast changing. Even specialties like obstetrics and gynaecology, which until recently reduced national training numbers, are now actively looking for recruits. The New Deal and the European Working Time Directive, which are discussed in Chapter 2, have massive implications for the number of doctors needed to run the existing service. Other factors, such as the increasing numbers of medical graduates who wish to take career breaks or work flexibly, also increase the opportunities for international doctors.

We have written a separate chapter on general practice for a number of reasons. First, general practitioners (GPs) are a huge entity. Second, this is one specialty that has traditionally provided worthwhile careers for international graduates; related to this is the fact that the generation of graduates who came here in the 1960s and 1970s are reaching retirement age, so there is an additional shortage in this field. Other healthcare systems do not have a primary care system at the centre of their service, so a full overview is given.

Throughout this book we have indicated the actual exam fees for college membership, and the price of a particular train ticket or a loaf of bread. These are only guidelines. As far as possible, they are accurate at the time the book went to press. However, it follows that exam fees will increase with the passage of time, as will the price of food and the cost of travel.

Doctors can expect to spend less time at work than their predecessors. What they can do with that free time is explored in Chapter 8. If you are to forego sunshine and warmth, the company of family and friends, you might as well take advantage of the culture, non-vocational education and sporting facilities available here. Apart from anything else, international doctors who are happy here tend to be those who have become involved in their local communities.

Peter Cross
Sabina Dosani
August 2004

About the authors

Sabina Dosani MBBS MSc MRCPsych is a specialist registrar in child and adolescent psychiatry at the Maudsley Hospital, London. She graduated from St Bartholomew's in 1998 and trained as a psychiatrist at Guy's and St Thomas'. She studied anthropology as part of an MSc at King's College, London. Sabina also works as a medical journalist and to date has had over 60 features, articles and reviews published in *Hospital Doctor, BMJ, Student BMJ, BMJ Careers, BMA News* and *Trauma*. As part of an internship at *The Guardian*, her work appeared in 'The Editor' section.

Peter Cross is a writer and journalist. Over 200 of his articles, features and book reviews have been published in the *Daily Telegraph, The Times*, the *Daily* and *Sunday Express* and the *Independent on Sunday*, where he wrote a weekly interview column entitled 'Nine to Five'. In 2002 his books, *Earning a Crust* and *Jobs for the Boys*, were published by Management Books 2000. He has written extensively for the medical and nursing press and is a regular contributor to the *Nursing Standard, Nursing Times, BMJ Careers* and *Student BMJ*. Peter teaches medical journalism and essay-writing skills to medical students at St Bartholomew's and the London School of Medicine and Dentistry.

Both authors are mixed-race second generation migrants. This is their third joint book.

Acknowledgements

We are grateful for the time, generosity and thoughtfulness of all the people who have helped with this book. Topics have been discussed with hundreds of international doctors, as well as with colleagues and friends – alas, too many to mention all by name.

Rhona MacDonald has been a source of inspiration to us both. She first drew our attention to the struggles and hurdles that international doctors face. Yong Lok Ong and Umesh Prabhu have been exceptionally generous in their encouragement and helpful advice, introducing us to ideas and concepts we would otherwise have missed. We are grateful to Arif Dosani for his perceptive comments on the section about money. Shehnaz Somjee kindly wrote detailed answers to our questions and the section on locums contains many of her opinions and advice.

We are grateful to the BMJ Publishing Group for allowing us to reproduce a series of articles on how to pass membership exams, first published in *BMJ Careers* in 2004. The BMJ Publishing Group also gave us permission to expand an article on death certificates that Sabina wrote for *Student BMJ*. Likewise, we thank RBI-UK (Reed Business International) for allowing us to base parts of this book on articles Sabina originally published in *Hospital Doctor* magazine.

The international doctors, who discussed so many topics with us, have affected this book more than anyone else. Many details have changed as a result of their comments and their enthusiasm turned what could have been a chore into a labour of love.

This book is dedicated to Dr Rhona MacDonald, GP, editor and long-distance runner – someone always prepared to go the extra mile.

CHAPTER 1

Before leaving home

Mid pleasures and palaces though we may roam,
Be it ever so humble, there's no place like home.

John Howard Payne (1791–1852)

A man's homeland is wherever he prospers.

Aristophanes (450 BC–388 BC)

■ Expectations

Doctors need to know what to expect when they come here. Not only PLAB exams and jobs, but also things like communicating with patients, taking a detailed history and how to involve relatives and a team.

Umesh Prabhu, consultant paediatrician from India

Most overseas doctors have a sense of disappointment. Everything takes time.

Anuga Shedeo, PLAB candidate

Moving to another country is a decision that should not be taken lightly. There are huge implications, not only for you but for other members of your family who may wish to see you at times other than your visits home. Below is a list of questions that anyone wishing to work in the UK should consider. You may have other questions specific to your circumstances. Time spent weighing up these arguments may not prevent you from making a wrong choice, nor experiencing the unexpected, but we suggest it will be time well spent. If possible, speak to someone who has migrated to the UK from your locality so you can benefit from their experiences and insights. This book will help you address these and other questions:

- What do I hope to gain by working as a doctor in Britain?
- What is the best stage of my career to work abroad?
- What is the best time of year for me to go?
- Who do I need to contact?
- Are my qualifications recognised or will I have to study for additional exams before I can work?
- What will it be like to leave family and close friends behind?
- What will I miss about my current job and life?
- Can I speak medical English?

- What do I know about British culture and what will it be like living there?
- Are there any visa requirements or restrictions?
- Where will I live when I get there?
- What can I do if I encounter racism ?

> I miss easy access to beaches. I miss really good supermarkets. There is a lot of processed food here and the fruit and vegetables are fresher at home. I miss open spaces and the sports culture we have in New Zealand.
> Stephanie Young, SpR psychiatrist from New Zealand

■ Essentials for training in the UK

Do you have:

- a valid passport
- UK entry clearance
- exemption from PLAB or proof of passing PLAB
- a primary medical qualification accepted by the GMC
- GMC registration
- a minimum of one year's post-qualification experience equivalent to that of a pre-registration house officer
- immunity to hepatitis B and a certificate proving this.

If you can answer yes to these questions, you can apply for training placements. If you still need to pass the Professional Linguistic Assessment Board (PLAB) examination, you can come to the UK on a visitor's visa, study for PLAB, undertake a clinical attachment, gain experience of the NHS and apply for a training post while on the clinical attachment.

It is worth getting your hepatitis B status checked before you leave. You will not be allowed to practise unless you have documented proof of hepatitis B immunity; thus if your UK entry clearance is dependent on you working as a doctor, you could be sent home.

■ Visas, work permits and permit-free training *(see Figure 1.1 on p. 5)*

European Economic Area (EEA) nationals (see Box 1.1) do not need a work permit and may work in the UK at any time.

Box 1.1 EEA countries

Austria	Latvia
Belgium	Liechtenstein
Cyprus	Lithuania
Czech Republic	Luxembourg
Denmark	Malta
Estonia	Netherlands
Finland	Norway
France	Poland
Germany	Portugal
Greece	Slovenia
Hungary	Spain
Iceland	Sweden
Ireland	Switzerland*
Italy	United Kingdom

*Switzerland is not an EEA country but a bi-lateral agreement with the EU means it is treated as if it were.

Visitor's visa

Doctors who are not EC nationals can come to the UK on a visitor's visa. This is valid for a stay of up to six months. In some cases an extension is allowed for a further six months. You are not allowed to work on this visa, but it is useful if you are doing the PLAB examination (*see* Chapter 6) or a clinical attachment (*see* Chapter 3). It is also useful if you are not yet registered with the GMC. If you enter the UK on a visitor's visa, you can apply for a *permit-free training* visa or a *work permit*.

Non-EC nationals can work in the UK under one of the following categories.

■ Certificate of Entitlement to Right of Abode

If you are a Commonwealth citizen and a British citizen by birth, adoption or registration, and descended from a father or mother or both in the UK, you will be eligible to work in the UK for an unlimited time.

■ Passport and Grandparent Entry Certificate

If one or both of your parents were born in the UK, you may be eligible for a British passport. Alternatively, if you have a British-born grandparent, you can apply for a UK Grandparent Entry Certificate which allows you to stay for up to four years.

If neither option applies, you need either a *work permit* or a *permit-free training* visa.

■ Work permit

Doctors with work permits are only eligible to work in a specific non-training post. Non-training posts are consultant, staff grade, associate specialist, or non-standard training grades. For information about the different types of posts, see Chapter 3. You are not able to work in pre-registration house officer (PRHO), senior house officer (SHO) or specialist registrar (SpR) posts. You usually need full GMC registration. This permit is not transferable between non-training posts. After four years, holders can apply for 'settled status'.

■ Permit-free training

> I did SHO training on permit-free training and they extended it for SpR training. The hassle is that you have to pay to get your visa renewed. It's over £100 and it used to be free. If you go in person it costs more than if you post it.
>
> Stephanie Young, SpR psychiatrist from New Zealand

This visa is for doctors who are applying for a recognised postgraduate training post: PRHO, SHO or SpR. Permit-free training is granted to doctors who intend to leave Britain at the end of their training and are eligible for GMC registration. It is usually limited to four years at SHO grade. The only exception to extension at SHO level is if you are appointed to a GP vocational training scheme (VTS, see Chapter 4). You will be able to stay on permit-free training for the duration of the VTS. If you are appointed to higher specialist training (type 1 or type 2 SpR, see Chapter 3) at the end of four years, your permit-free training can be extended. It will be issued for the length of your job contract.

> People who have not reached their training goals will have to try to get a LAT [locum appointment for training] or LAS [locum appointment for service] and extend their permit-free training that way. Permit-free training is a ticking clock. If for any reason you have to come off training posts for personal or professional reasons, come off permit-free training. Apply to stay on a visitor's visa to stop that clock. If you are married to another overseas doctor, you have four years permit-free training each. Use each lot consecutively and you get eight years.
>
> Yong Lok Ong, consultant old age psychiatrist from
> Singapore and Overseas Doctors' Dean, London Deanery

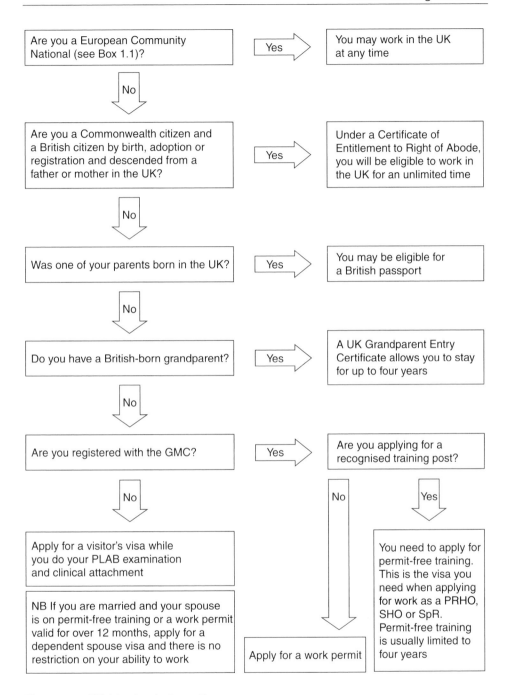

Figure 1.1   Which visa do I need?

■ Getting registered with the GMC

I didn't know it would take so long to get registered with the GMC. If you need PLAB, do part 1 at home, then come here to do part 2 and apply for jobs.

Blessing Dhwayo, doctor from Zimbabwe

■ The General Medical Council

The GMC was established under the auspices of the Medical Act 1858 and maintains the register of medical practitioners and the register of medical practitioners with limited registration. As well as maintaining these registers, the GMC also promotes good medical practice, sets standards, administers PLAB, and handles complaints and concerns about doctors accused of not being fit to practise. It is able to take a range of actions from warning a doctor about poor performance to (in serious cases) removing their name from the register. More recently the GMC has taken on the role of revalidation. This means that from 2005 doctors will be given a licence to practise medicine and, to maintain this licence, they must take part in revalidation when asked to do so by the GMC. To keep a licence each doctor will need to demonstrate that they have been practising according to the standards set out in *Good Medical Practice*,[1] described in Box 1.2. It is anticipated that revalidation will take place every five years. See the GMC website www.gmc-uk.org for further information.

Box 1.2 Duties of a doctor registered with the General Medical Council

'Patients must be able to trust doctors with their lives and wellbeing. To justify that trust, we as a profession have a duty to maintain a good standard of practice and care and to show respect for human life. In particular, as a doctor you must:

- make the care of your patient your first concern
- treat every patient politely and considerately
- respect patients' dignity and privacy
- listen to patients and respect their views
- give patients information in a way they can understand
- respect the rights of patients to be fully involved in decisions about their care
- keep your professional knowledge and skills up to date
- recognise the limits of your professional competence
- be honest and trustworthy
- respect and protect confidential information
- make sure that your personal beliefs do not prejudice your patients' care
- act quickly to protect patients from risk if you have good reason to believe that you or a colleague may not be fit to practise
- avoid abusing your position as a doctor
- work with colleagues in the ways that best serve patients' interests.'

For doctors graduating outside the UK there are a number of different paths to GMC registration. The process generally depends on where you obtained your primary medical qualification and your nationality.

Doctors who are nationals of and qualify in an EEA member state (*see* Box 1.1) (or non-EEA nationals with European Community [EC] rights) are eligible for full registration. They can also apply for provisional registration if their medical education includes a period of postgraduate clinical training (internship training). Doctors qualifying in Switzerland and who are EEA nationals (or non-EEA nationals with EC rights) or Swiss nationals are also eligible for full registration. This also applies to Swiss nationals who have qualified in another EEA member state.

At present there are three types of GMC registration – provisional, limited and full – but this is due to change in 2005 (*see* below). However, you don't need to be registered with the GMC for a clinical attachment (*see* Chapter 3).

Provisional registration

Provisional registration allows newly qualified doctors from the UK or EEA to undertake general clinical training under supervision, which is needed for full registration. A doctor who is provisionally registered is entitled to work only in resident PRHO posts in hospitals or institutions that are approved for the purpose of PRHO service.

Limited registration

Limited registration is granted to overseas doctors and some from the EEA for employment in a specific recognised training post, approved by the relevant Royal College and supervised by a registered medical practitioner. Doctors applying for limited registration need to check they have a primary medical qualification that the GMC accepts. Over 1600 overseas primary medical qualifications are accepted by the GMC. They include all the primary medical qualifications listed in the *World Directory of Medical Schools*,[2] published by the World Health Organization (WHO),* and a number of others listed on the GMC website. All applicants for limited registration must demonstrate their suitability to practise in the UK. You can do this by passing the PLAB examination. Limited registration is granted for up to five years of training. There may be restrictions on the grade and/or specialty you can work in.

To be eligible for limited registration you need three things:

1 a primary medical qualification recognised by the GMC
2 a minimum of one year's experience in a PRHO equivalent or intern post
3 to pass or be exempt from the PLAB examination.

Full registration

You need full registration for unsupervised medical practice in the NHS or private practice in the UK. You may also need specialist registration if you wish to take up a substantive, honorary or fixed term consultant post (other than a locum consultant post) within the NHS.

From 2005, limited registration will be abolished and replaced with a single licensing system covering all doctors, irrespective of whether they have qualified in the UK, EEA or elsewhere. We strongly recommend you stay updated through the GMC website: www.gmc-uk.org/register/consultation_paper/.

---

* Except those in traditional Chinese medicine or American qualifications in osteopathy.

The main changes under the proposed new system are:

- a single licensing structure will apply to all doctors, regardless of where they have qualified
- no separate probationary system for overseas qualified doctors
- principles governing eligibility for a licence will be the same for all doctors
- doctors will not have to secure employment in order to obtain a licence
- all doctors will be required to revalidate within two years of being awarded their first general licence
- prior to their first revalidation, doctors will be required to limit their practice to work in a managed environment
- before a doctor can lose a general licence, the GMC will need to demonstrate that they are not fit to practise.

This differs from the current regime for non-EEA qualified doctors who are required to demonstrate their suitability to practise every time they renew their limited registration and when they apply to move from limited to full registration.

■ The Overseas Doctors Training Scheme

The Overseas Doctors Training Scheme (ODTS) is a sponsorship scheme set up by the Department of Health (DoH) and the Royal Colleges, but administered by the relevant Royal College. Royal Colleges arrange for sponsored doctors to be granted limited GMC registration and exemption from PLAB.

The ODTS provides postgraduate training posts to high-calibre, overseas-qualified doctors so that they can continue or complete specialist training before returning to a specialist career at home. It is not intended that overseas doctors remain in the UK on completion of their specialist training. Every Royal College has its own ODTS policy, outlined below. Sponsorship provides objective evidence of applicants' capability.

Sponsored trainees are subject to the conditions for leave to enter from the Immigration Office. Conditions of this leave are stamped in passports. The Royal College will provide the necessary documentation for trainees to obtain a permit-free training visa and passport stamp.

Sponsorship restricts ODTS doctors to a specific Royal College and GMC-approved post. Once you are on the ODTS you cannot work outside your sponsorship arrangement. Royal Colleges deal with the GMC on the candidate's behalf. Applicants must have a primary medical qualification which is acceptable for limited GMC registration. Royal Colleges check this. Shortly before a doctor arrives in the UK, the Royal College will ask for original primary medical qualification certificates and an International English Language Testing System (IELTS) certificate for the GMC. ODTS doctors are registered with the GMC for no more than 12 months in the first instance. This may be extended if the Postgraduate Dean and Royal College recommend it, and is dependent on satisfactory progress and availability of suitable posts.

Overseas doctors must have passed the academic version of the IELTS (*see* Chapter 6) to be granted limited registration. This includes doctors from

English-speaking countries: the USA, Australia, New Zealand, Canada, South Africa and the Caribbean.

Doctors who meet any of the following criteria are also excluded from applying for the ODTS:

- those who have previously failed the PLAB examination
- those who qualified in and/or who are nationals of an EEA country, or those with enforceable EC rights
- those who are already working or resident in the UK, or another member state of the EEA.

■ Royal College ODTS policies

Royal College of Anaesthetists

The initial approach must be made by a UK consultant or senior lecturer. All appointments must be to substantive, approved training posts.

Royal College of Obstetricians and Gynaecologists

This College runs an 'Overseas Training Fellowship Scheme'. In essence, this is two years at specialist registrar grade. All applicants must meet the following criteria:

- must have passed part 1 of the MRCOG (Member of the Royal College of Obstetrics and Gynaecology) examination or equivalent by recognised exemption
- must have passed the IELTS examination at the approved level with at least 12 months remaining at the time of application
- three years of supervised practice in obstetrics and gynaecology
- be currently domiciled in their home country
- have not previously registered with the UK General Medical Council.

An application pack can be downloaded from the College website: www.rcog.org.uk

Royal College of Ophthalmologists

All posts must be approved for training by the College and Postgraduate Dean.

Enquiries may be emailed to education@rcophth.btinternet.com. Information is also available on the College's website: www.rcophth.ac.uk.

Royal College of Paediatrics and Child Health

The 'International Paediatric Training Scheme' (IPTS) is used here. Doctors work in SHO posts and are eligible for up to four years of permit-free training.

All applicants must:

- have completed a minimum of three years' paediatric clinical experience overseas
- have completed an acceptable internship of not less than 12 months
- have passed the final qualifying examination for a primary medical qualification accepted by the GMC for limited registration
- hold non-EU citizenship (exceptions will be made for doctors with refugee status) and be living outside the EU

- be proposed to the College by their current overseas consultant, who must be willing to act as the applicant's overseas sponsor and be in a position to state that the applicant will be eligible for re-employment on completion of training in the UK
- have achieved a minimum score of 7.0 in each of the four bands of the IELTS examination.

Royal College of Physicians and Surgeons of Glasgow

The initial approach to the College should be made by the UK sponsor. An overseas sponsor is also required. The UK training post must be a salaried substantive NHS training post carrying both educational approval and approval by the Postgraduate Dean.

Appointments must be arranged in the UK before application for the ODTS is submitted. The College is not able to arrange training posts for sponsored doctors at the time of writing.

Royal College of Physicians of Edinburgh

The College has currently suspended the Overseas Doctors Training Scheme. You are advised to contact them direct for updated information.

Royal College of Physicians of London

The ODTS is closed at present. Email international@rcplondon.ac.uk for updated information.

Royal College of Psychiatrists

The ODTS has been closed permanently. However, the College operates a 'Consultant-Assisted Sponsorship Scheme'. Applicants must have a UK sponsor who should be an NHS consultant and a Member of the Royal College of Psychiatrists. The initial application should be made by the UK sponsor who must be able to offer the applicant a fully approved training post within their own training scheme. The UK sponsor must also provide written confirmation that they know the overseas sponsor personally.

Royal College of Radiologists

The Royal College of Radiologists does not operate an ODTS.

Royal College of Surgeons of Edinburgh

It is the responsibility of the overseas sponsor to set up a post for the applicant in the UK, in partnership with a UK consultant. The UK consultant offering the post then makes contact with the College on behalf of the overseas applicant.

Royal College of Surgeons of England

Applicants must be nominated by an approved sponsoring body in their home country. The Royal College of Surgeons of England, rather than an individual surgeon, acts as the UK sponsoring body. The College is not able to arrange training posts for sponsored doctors. It only sponsors trainees for higher surgical training posts, and applicants must have an appointment arranged in the UK before applying for the College ODTS.

■ Four golden rules for the ODTS

1 *Do* contact the relevant Royal College directly for their most up-to-date ODTS policy. Follow their instructions to the letter.
2 *Do* expect to pay an administration fee of around £500.
3 *Don't* apply directly to a Royal College; only appropriate sponsors may apply on your behalf.
4 *Don't* be disheartened. Many more applications are received than there are training posts available.

Packing

If you are coming to the UK from a country where the cost of living is lower, it is worth bringing a range of suitable outfits with you rather than having to purchase new, expensive clothes when you arrive. However, some items such as umbrellas are cheaper to purchase in the UK. British medical staff dress in a formal manner so men will need a selection of shirts and ties and women a range of smart, modest attire.

The British climate varies but generally autumn and winter (September to March) can be cold and damp with temperatures falling below freezing between December and February. Anticipate wind, rain, frost and snow and pack accordingly. If you are going to be in the UK in winter you will need jumpers, a fleece jacket, raincoat, waterproof shoes and an umbrella. On the other hand, summer can be hot and you will be able to spend more time outdoors.

We recommend all international doctors bring:

- at least £250 cash for room key deposits, swipe card, parking permit, taxi fares, meals and other miscellaneous expenses
- traveller's cheques
- ten passport photographs for identification (ID) cards, e.g. for the library, exam entry, etc.

■ References

1 General Medical Council (2001) *Good Medical Practice*. GMC, London.

2 World Health Organization (2000) *The World Directory of Medical Schools*: www.who. int/en/

CHAPTER 2

Medicine in Britain

The British have no unifying faith, only a belief in the National Health Service.

Nigel Lawson (1932–), former Chancellor of the Exchequer

■ Understanding the NHS

No matter what you hear on television, this is one of the best health systems in the world. It is free at the point of delivery and there is great commitment, concern, honesty and integrity of care.

Samja Mishra, SHO in ophthalmology from India

The British National Health Service (NHS) is one of the wonders of the world. It is the third largest employer on the planet. The only two organisations employing more staff are the Chinese Red Army and the Indian Railway.

Health was one of many social reforms that were conceived during the Second World War when there was a lot of thought about the sort of society Britain should have once Hitler had been removed. The NHS was thus created by an ambitious Labour Government in 1948. We would argue that time spent understanding something about the early days of the NHS, its subsequent history and attempted reforms helps prospective employees understand the vast organisation it has become. The founding fathers and their supporters anticipated that the health benefits of a nationalised rather than private health service would lead to a healthier population and decreased demand. This logic led them to believe that the service would shrink, becoming progressively less expensive to run. They would soon discover that the reverse was true. Demand and expectations have always exceeded the funding that governments were able or willing to provide.

It is worth noting that the medical establishment was initially sceptical, fearing an adverse effect on its members' incomes, and a number of concessions had to be made to get this powerful group on board. Since then the profession's contribution has been mixed: reactionary and progressive, altruistic and self-interested in an ongoing power struggle with non-medical managers and politicians.

Insufficient funding and ideological differences have ensured that this lumbering giant has staggered from crisis to crisis, malnourished on insufficient taxpayers' money, too big and inflexible to adapt to changing needs. Yet somehow it has been able to survive, in part due to memories of pre-war insecurity and a popular endorsement by the general public, and also by a failure to come up with anything better.

It could be argued that the service has survived due to a pragmatic and dedicated workforce, particularly apparent in the so-called Cinderella specialties like psychiatry, old age medicine and family planning that are heavily reliant on the contribution of overseas doctors who are pleased to work in the UK, hoping to make a better life for themselves and their families.

■ Then and now

The NHS is financed through taxes. Almost everyone has access to a general practitioner (GP) who makes specialist referrals when necessary.

UK healthcare before the NHS was very different (*see* Figure 2.1). Hospitals were mainly used by the poor, and there were major financial barriers to healthcare for many people. Consultants' income came from private practice and the work they did in hospitals was for free. Specialists and GPs were unevenly distributed nationally and medical care was uncoordinated. GPs were not able to admit patients to hospital.

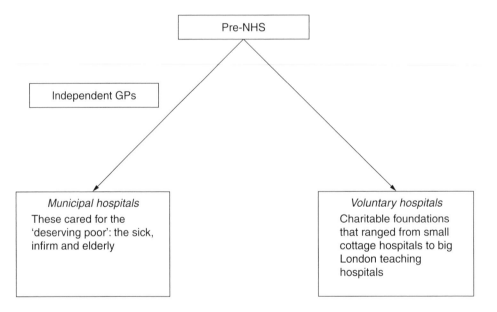

Figure 2.1 Healthcare in Britain before the NHS.

During the Second World War, civil servant William Henry Beveridge produced a blueprint for postwar reconstruction. In 1942 the Beveridge Report identified 'five giants':

1 want
2 disease
3 ignorance
4 squalor
5 indolence.

Beveridge recommended a *welfare state* which was to include:

- universal healthcare
- retirement pensions for all
- provision for dependent children.

The medical profession resisted these proposals. GPs felt a salaried service would threaten their professional autonomy and consultants were worried about their pay in the NHS.

In 1946, the Labour Health Minister, Aneurin Bevan, proposed a solution. He opted for a regional rather than local scheme with executive control over municipal and voluntary hospitals. Under the NHS Act 1946, GPs remained independent contractors but were better off financially and hospital consultants were paid for hospital work that they had previously done for free. They were also allowed to keep private practices. Merit awards were introduced for hospital consultants. However, in 1948 it transpired that costs had been underestimated and so ceiling expenditure was imposed. A theme of underfunding has stayed with the NHS to the present day.

In 1962 there was a consensus that the NHS needed reform. Conservative Minister for Health, Enoch Powell, pioneered the 1962 Hospital Plan. Powell set up district general hospitals with 600–800 beds to serve population districts of 100 000, to allow for better allocation of scarce resources. He was also influential in recruiting medical and nursing personnel from overseas.

Staffing levels were critically low in the 1960s. Many doctors left and went to the USA. More medical schools were founded to address this shortfall and doctors were paid more to try to prevent them leaving. Doctors were also getting stuck at senior registrar grade, some spending as long as 15 years waiting for consultant posts. The senior registrar grade was restricted to match consultant vacancies and the medical assistant grade was introduced.

In 1974 the NHS was reformed again. It remained accountable to the Government, but below the Department of Health and Social Security were regional health authorities (RHAs). These authorities allocated money and monitored area health authorities (AHAs). Short- and long-term goals were set by region, area and district. GPs were still independent contractors. The 1974 reforms resulted in a 30% increase in NHS administrators. Inequalities in provision prevailed. Building programmes were axed in an attempt to cut costs.

Roy Griffiths, Chairman of Sainsbury's supermarket (*see* Chapter 8), was invited to undertake a further review of NHS management in 1983. He made four key recommendations:

1 there should be a general manager in charge at each level
2 decentralise decision making
3 involve clinicians in decision making
4 strengthen power at regional level.

The 1980s saw other changes. Project 2000 was introduced in 1988. This represented a new era in nurse training, where nurses studied for academic qualifications to diploma and degree level and were perceived as 'knowledgeable doers'. The 1987 report *Hospital Medical Staffing: Achieving a Balance*[1] responded to the crisis in consultant numbers by increasing them, restricting numbers of training-grade doctors (*see* Chapter 3) and introducing the staff grade (*see* Chapter 3).

The NHS was still suffering from chronic underfunding. In 1989 the Conservative Government responded to the funding crisis with the White Paper *Working for Patients*.[2] A 'provider market' was introduced, based on separation of districts as purchasers and NHS units as providers. This was designed to stimulate competition and create an internal market in the NHS as a cure for inefficiency.

In 1991 the Conservative Government produced another White Paper, *The Health of the Nation*,[3] which identified five key areas to prevent untimely deaths:

- coronary heart disease
- cancer
- HIV/AIDS
- mental illness
- accidents.

The Calman Report in 1993[4] merged the registrar and senior registrar grades and reduced specialist training to seven years. Explicit criteria leading to a Certificate of Completion of Specialist Training (CCST) were introduced.

In 1997 there was a change of Government and the Labour Party returned to power. The Department of Health consultation document *Unfinished Business* was published in 2002.[5] It is the Government's proposed reform to the SHO grade, and includes a plan to turn the PRHO year into a two-year foundation programme. It encourages exposure to different specialties, informed career advice and proper assessments. It proposes two phases of SHO education and training and emphasises five main points about its implementation, saying that it should:

- be programme-based
- be broadly based to begin with for all trainees
- have individually tailored programmes to meet special needs
- be time-limited.

In October 2003 a new consultant contract was introduced. All consultants appointed after this date automatically work under the new contract. Existing consultants are able to choose whether to remain on their previous contract or move to the new one. A major advantage of the new contract is that it provides an explicit description of what consultants do each day. Agreeing a job plan is an integral part of the new contract, which consists of ten programmed activities, each lasting four hours (three in premium time outside 7am–7pm, Monday to Friday). The working week includes:

- direct clinical care and travelling time
- supporting professional activities, including audit, research, continuing professional development and teaching others
- additional NHS responsibilities, for example medical director, clinical tutor, postgraduate dean
- external duties such as BMA work.

Consultants can expect to earn a minimum of £63 000, roughly £10 000 more than under the old contract. The new contract puts a 40-hour limit on the basic working week, as the BMA complained that most consultants were regularly working a 50-hour NHS week.

■ Types of hospital

> UK hospitals are different from ones back home. Here there is meticulous patient care and excellent management.
>
> Prashamt Borade, doctor from India

There are a number of different types of hospital employing doctors in the UK. There are also places like cottage hospitals, old people's homes and sheltered accommodation where GPs and other medical staff may visit and see more than one patient, but they have not been included here as we are more concerned with describing establishments where doctors are based for most of their working week.

The main types of hospitals providing employment for doctors are as follows.

■ Teaching hospitals

Teaching hospitals are usually the main hospitals in university towns and cities. The university employs consultants and other senior medical staff, who hold 'honorary' contracts with the NHS trust. Teaching hospitals care for patients with complex or rare conditions. Many are centres of excellence for particular conditions, for example in oncology or cardiology.

■ District general hospitals

These are regional hospitals that treat patients with a range of common conditions. Patients with complex or rare conditions are usually referred to teaching hospitals. The NHS employs all medical staff.

■ Psychiatric hospitals

Psychiatric patients have been provided with specialist institutions in the UK for many hundreds of years. During the late nineteenth century, many large establishments were built for the mentally ill and for patients with what is now called learning disabilities. Some of these large establishments still exist, but only care for a fraction of the patients they once did. Psychiatric units attached to district general hospitals have largely replaced separate psychiatric hospitals. This places patients nearer to their local communities and means that patients and psychiatrists have easier access to services like phlebotomy, scans and medical opinions.

■ Prison hospitals

Many of Britain's prisons have hospital wings.

■ Military hospitals

While not as numerous as in earlier decades, Britain's armed services have hospital facilities for servicemen and women. Medical provision is usually by medical officers, but civilian doctors sometimes make up the shortfall.

■ Private hospitals

For information about private hospitals, *see* 'Resident medical officers in the private sector' in Chapter 3 (p. 38).

■ Teamwork

> Many overseas doctors are not used to multidisciplinary teamworking. They still think doctors are on top of the pyramid. They meet a senior nurse consultant and are thrown.
>
> Yong Lok Ong, consultant old age psychiatrist from Singapore and Overseas Doctors Dean, London Deanery

> I had been here a week when I was told I was the rudest doctor in the hospital because I never said please or thank you to the nurses. I learnt how powerful nurses are. The consultant always asks them how good the doctor is. The senior nurse from the special care baby unit put in a good word for me with the consultant and that helped me get my job. In India, nurses are looked down on. I had to learn about teamwork.
>
> Umesh Prabhu, consultant paediatrician from India

In the UK most doctors work in teams with other doctors and other healthcare professionals. Within hospitals, doctors work in multi-professional teams that include medical staff, nurses, physiotherapists, occupational therapists, psychologists, other healthcare workers and technicians. There are a number of advantages of multi-professional teamwork: professionals from various backgrounds, ethnic groups, age ranges and training bring a wider range of skills, knowledge and life experiences than any one individual (*see* Box 2.1). The whole is greater than the constituent parts. Patients have access to a wider range of skills, better continuity of care and greater flexibility.

Box 2.1 Essential characteristics of teamwork[3]

- Members share a common purpose, which binds them together and guides their actions.
- Each team member has a clear understanding of their functions and recognises common interests.
- Teamwork progresses by pooling knowledge, skills and resources.
- All members share responsibility for outcome.

British hospitals are complex organisms. Lay people tend to assume unthinkingly that they are staffed almost entirely by doctors and nurses and, if pushed, may concede that these places also employ cooks, cleaners and porters. In fact, hospitals directly or indirectly employ a vast array of front-line and support staff who work behind the scenes. For example, paramedics do much more than simply collecting patients and ferrying them to hospital. Many are experts in resuscitation and provide life-saving care on the way to hospital. Hospital pharmacists visit wards and review prescription charts. They often contact junior doctors to discuss drug choices, doses and other therapeutic options. Many attend and contribute to ward rounds.

All patients admitted to hospital are under a named consultant's care. Inpatients are usually assigned a 'named nurse'. A number of doctors who have trained over-seas have told us how much British nurses differ from those they have worked with before.

British nurses do not see themselves as 'the doctor's handmaiden' and generally resent being used as a servant. They are autonomous professionals. Ward sisters and managers are usually assertive and, while respectful of medical training and expertise, can be vocal about doctors who they feel fall below what they consider an acceptable standard.

Many nurses have diverse clinical skills, including phlebotomy, ECG inter-pretation and intravenous drug administration. Some nurses have an extended role, sharing core skills once exclusively carried out by doctors, for example endoscopy, deliberate self-harm assessment and palliative care.

■ What makes a good team?

What makes a good team will vary according to different circumstances. The dynamics and qualities needed for a surgical team will differ from a team charged with caring for terminally ill cancer patients. Having said that, most would agree that good teams have the following traits:

- *Good leadership.* Leadership need not only be provided by the most senior members of the team, it can come from other experienced staff, colleagues with a strong commitment and non-medical team players.
- *A democratic culture.* While it is true that in certain circumstances strong auto-cratic leadership is called for, good teams take account of creative suggestions, thoughts and feelings of all their members and are prepared to modify actions in the light of democratic discussions.
- *Shared goals and values.* Members of strong and successful teams tend to have unified aims and objectives that are more important than individual differences of class, creed, race, gender and so on.
- *A commitment to learning and training.* Good teams are keen to learn from experiences, good and bad, sharing outcomes and finding ways of improving practice. This can only be achieved in a no-blame culture where there is a will-ingness for individuals and teams to take responsibility for mishaps and mistakes.
- *Mutual respect and support.* Good teams are made up of players who are aware of the importance of colleagues and qualities others have that they lack them-selves, i.e. other's skills, training and experiences; an awareness that the whole team is greater than the sum of the individual players.

• *Openness to outsiders*. The best teams are friendly, warm and accessible to new members and outsiders, with a willingness to consider, learn and adapt existing practice. Good teams never seem smug or self-satisfied.

■ When teams go wrong

Replacing an autocratic style of service delivery with something more democratic can lead to procrastination, rivalry, compromise, lack of leadership and staff working beyond their sphere of expertise (*see* Box 2.2).

Box 2.2 Potential disadvantages of multi-professional work[7]

• *Communication problems* – these arise when team members omit to inform colleagues of developments in a patient's need or care.
• *Competition* – interprofessional rivalry occurs if there is considerable overlap between fields of activity.
• *Duplication* – this is wasteful of resources and may result in conflicting messages being given to patients.

Multi-professional teams function best where there is strong altruistic leadership. This need not necessarily be provided by a medical figurehead – for instance a consultant – but could be a ward manager. The role of the leader is to ensure that individuals remain focused on team goals and feel valued and respected for what they have to offer. The best teams bring out qualities in individuals that would not be utilised anywhere else.

■ The British Medical Association (BMA)

Sir Charles Hastings (1794–1866) founded the British Medical Association in 1832. From the outset the Association struggled for medical reform. After 20 years of negotiation, the 1858 Medical Act was included in the statute-book. The Act established the General Medical Council and the Medical Register, therefore distinguishing, for the first time, qualified from unqualified practitioners.

The BMA is the doctors' trade union and professional association. Although membership is not compulsory, 80% of UK doctors join. BMA activities include negotiating doctors' national terms and conditions, providing representation in disciplinary hearings and presenting doctors' views to the Government of the day. The BMA also offers a range of services, from organising loans and insurance at preferential rates to running a wine-tasting club and a free counselling helpline.

■ Royal Colleges

The Royal Colleges are independent professional bodies governed by councils that are elected by members. Membership of a Royal College is obtained by examination and is essential for specialist hospital practice in the NHS. Some Colleges, like the Royal College of Physicians, are hundreds of years old, while others, like the Royal College of General Practitioners, were founded recently.

Royal Colleges set standards of knowledge, skills and experience that are needed for specialist training and career progression in their specialty. They produce a syllabus of these requirements. Royal Colleges set and mark postgraduate examinations that may be for a diploma, or for membership of the College. Representatives of Royal Colleges inspect approved training posts, as they grant educational approval.

Membership exams are held regularly in the UK and in some cases overseas. Detailed information can be found in Chapter 6. A doctor's eligibility to sit an exam is decided by the relevant College.

■ The New Deal

Before the New Deal, junior doctors worked long hours – 120-hour weeks were common. GP and former barrister Sam Everington led the campaign to reduce these hours:

> I recognised this was awful but most junior doctors didn't. If you're working long hours you begin to think that this is a normal way of life. Yet research had shown 28% of junior doctors had evidence of depression and 50% were emotionally disturbed. Working long hours was dangerous for patients. I had done a number of pieces of media work before and wondered how we could make a difference. I got hold of a friend and we slept outside the London Hospital for 48 hours and got immense coverage. When journalists asked what my campaign was, I said it was to reduce our hours to 72 hours a week. There was a realisation that this was serious. I talked about how I and other doctors made mistakes. There was a doctor who had fallen asleep during an operation and woke up on top of the patient. David Mellor, Health Minister at the time, accused me of telling fisherman's tales, and so we produced the doctor. I issued a writ against the hospital for not ensuring health and safety at work, a breech of their common-law duty. It turned into a big campaign. We took it all the way to the House of Lords, and we won.

The BMA's Junior Doctors Committee agreed the New Deal.[8] This removed overtime pay, which was previously paid at a lower rate than normal hourly rates. From 1 August 2001, it became illegal for newly qualified doctors to work more than 56 hours per week, or without sufficient rest. The same limit applied to all other doctors from August 2003.

■ Pay banding

Since the New Deal, a junior doctor's salary consists of a basic salary to which a supplement, also known as a multiplier, is added. The supplement is calculated as a proportion of the basic salary according to the pay band to which the post is designated (*see* Box 2.3). For example, Dr Curtis' basic salary is £25 000 per annum. She is in band 2b. Therefore she will get £25 000, plus 50% of this, so will earn £37 500 before tax.

Box 2.3 Proportion of supplement (multiplier) according to pay band

Band	Multiplier
3	100%
2a	80%
2b	50%
1a	50%
1b	40%
1c	20%

■ The European Working Time Directive

The European Working Time Directive (EWTD) came into force on 1 October 1998 for consultants and other career-grade hospital doctors.[9] The Directive is being applied to junior doctors according to the timetable in Box 2.4.

Box 2.4 EWTD timetable

August 2004 – interim 58-hour maximum working week. Rest and break requirements become law.
August 2007 – interim 56-hour maximum working week.
August 2009 – deadline for 48-hour maximum working week.

The EWTD also stipulates rest requirements, which are detailed in Box 2.5.

Box 2.5 EWTD rest requirements

The rest requirements, which came into effect in August 2004, are:

- a minimum daily consecutive period of 11 hours
- a minimum rest break of 20 minutes when the working day exceeds six hours
- a minimum rest period of 24 hours in each seven-day period (this can be averaged to be a 40-hour rest period in 14 days)
- a minimum of four weeks' paid annual leave
- a maximum of eight hours work in each 24 hours for night workers.

■ The SIMAP case

In 2000, the European Court of Justice (ECJ), in a case concerning primary care doctors in Spain (the SIMAP case), ruled that all time resident on-call was work.[10] This ruling will also apply to doctors in training in the UK. Therefore, from August 2004, the New Deal's 72-hour limit for doctors resident on-call must be reduced to 58 hours per week.

■ Clinical governance

Until quite recently quality in the NHS varied enormously. Now, each health authority has a duty to maintain standards and improve quality through the introduction of clinical governance in 1998.

Clinical governance is the way that every health organisation will meet its duty of quality assurance. This means that NHS organisations are now accountable for continuously improving services and ensuring high standards of care. The chief executive is now accountable on behalf of the Board of each organisation.

Key components of clinical governance include:

- quality improvement
- continuing professional development
- it is evidence based
- audit
- risk reduction
- development of information strategies.

The National Institute for Clinical Excellence (NICE) sets standards and the Commission for Health Improvement (CHI) inspects local clinical governance arrangements. Individual practitioners are expected to take a greater part in audit, team leadership, appraisal, adopting NICE guidelines, involving service users in the planning of services and continuing professional development (CPD). Also, poor clinician performance should be recognised by early-detection mechanisms alongside revalidation of doctors every five years. It is hoped that the overall culture will be more open, participative and evaluative.

■ Medical slang and colloquialisms

Patients here know a lot about their diseases. Even more than the doctors sometimes.

Anand Sharma, SHO in internal medicine from India

When somebody told me about her water infection I thought the water in her house had got infected. Here water infection means kidney infection. In India if you are sick you are very ill; here it means you are vomiting.

Umesh Prabhu, consultant paediatrician from India

> My wife was working in Liverpool and she was pregnant at the time. One of the patients said, 'You must be "made up"'. For her 'made up' meant constipated, when the patient meant 'you must be happy'. This was the difference between Manchester and Liverpool.
>
> Professor Michael Cormi, British GP

English is a dynamic and ever-evolving language. This is especially true in medicine, which has its own rich tradition of dark humour to help practitioners cope with the bleak abnormalities of their everyday lives. It should be added that these remarks are merely coping mechanisms, throw-away comments meant for medical colleagues and certainly not for patients' or their relatives' ears or eyes. Terms like:

ash cash – money for signing a cremation form
bash cash – the money paid for completing claim forms
CABG (pronounced cabbage) – coronary artery bypass graft
coffin dodger – elderly patient
Freud squad – psychiatrists
gas men – anaesthetists
ISQ (in *status quo*) – no change
oligoneuronal – not very clever.

These terms should only be used with known colleagues and never written down, as patients may have access to their medical notes and could sue you for writing derogatory remarks.

> A little bit of advice: use words like *wonderful, brilliant, fantastic, great* and *lovely* instead of *good* or *yes*. But don't say 'Fantastic' if someone says 'My dad died of bowel cancer'.
>
> Tha Han, doctor from Myanmar

A fuller list of medical slang can be found at: www.shartwell.freeserve.co.uk/humor-site/medical-acronyms.htm.

Patients often use words and expressions that may not be familiar. Typically, a woman might tell you she is 'up the duff', 'has a bun in the oven', or is 'expecting'. A widow might inform you that her husband has 'gone to meet his maker', is 'six foot under', or 'has passed away'. All these terms suggest reluctance on the patient's part to use direct words like *pregnant* or *dead*.

Other patients will tell you that they have 'a frog in their throat', meaning it is sore, or have 'butterflies in their stomach' when they are nervous and agitated. If you do not understand such colloquialisms, ask for clarification.

The words and expressions that you may chance upon are likely to vary enormously and depend on such factors as the part of the country, age of the speaker, his or her gender, social class and other cultural influences. It is worth discussing this when being inducted in a new locality.

■ References

1 Department of Health (1987) *Hospital Medical Staffing: Achieving a Balance*. The Stationery Office, London.

2 Department of Health (1989) *Working for Patients*. The Stationery Office, London.

3 Department of Health (1991) *The Health of the Nation*. The Stationery Office, London.

4 Working Group on Specialist Medical Training (Calman Report) (1993) *Hospital Doctors: training for the future*. Department of Health, London.

5 Department of Health (2002) *Unfinished Business*. The Stationery Office, London. www.doh.gov.uk/shoconsult

6 Pritchard P (1981) *Manual of Primary Care: its nature and organization*. Oxford University Press, Oxford.

7 Jarman B (1988) *Primary Care*. Heinemann Medical Press, London.

8 NHS Management Executive (1991) *Junior Doctors: the new deal*. Department of Health, London.

9 MacDonald R (2003) Implementing the European Working Time Directive. *BMJ*. **327**: S9.

10 www.doh.gov.uk/workingtime/simap.htm

■ Further reading

Diamond J (1991) *C: because cowards get cancer too*. Vermillion, London.

Fox AT, Cahill P and Fertleman M (2002) Medical slang. *BMJ*. **324**: S179.

Swage T (2003) *Clinical Governance in Healthcare Practice*. Butterworth Heinemann, Oxford.

CHAPTER 3

Career planning

If you want to go back, go back within four years. After that you won't
settle. There is a gradual change in you that you won't notice.

Umesh Prabhu, consultant paediatrician from India

Fail to prepare, prepare to fail. We live in a competitive world and medicine is a
competitive profession. The people who become successful on their own terms are
not necessarily the brightest or the best, rather individuals who have looked at
themselves, assessed their strengths and weaknesses, likes and dislikes, and have
devised a career plan that takes account of their skills, potential and aspirations.
It also makes allowances for commitments and interests away from the workplace.

There is little formal career guidance for doctors working in the UK, but lots of
ad hoc tips, advice and suggestions from peers, consultants, tutors and deans. The
quality of this advice varies according to a number of factors: the wisdom and
experience of the person you are talking to, how objective they may be and, in this
fast-changing world, whether the information they give you is accurate. The wise
build on good counsel and reject rubbish. However helpful others' advice may
be, the best decisions are made by thinking through the issues. Here are a few
questions that you might consider:

- What do you hope to be doing in five years' time?
- What do you need to get out of your time in the UK to help you achieve your
  aim?
- What do you need to do now?
- Who do you know that can help you?
- How long do you plan to stay in the UK?
- What responsibilities do you have now and in the medium term?
- What are the implications for your family?

■ Choosing a specialty

You need to choose a specialty you are interested in and not compromise.
It is harder for international doctors in oversubscribed specialties, but not
impossible. You need to do twice as much. Do an audit early on. Try and
publish research early. Again, it is hard but not impossible. There are a lot
of successful international doctors in oversubscribed specialties. Be true to
yourself. We spend our whole lives working and if you are going to do something you are not keen on and if your heart isn't in it, you will be so unhappy.

Yong Lok Ong, consultant old age psychiatrist from
Singapore and Overseas Doctors Dean, London Deanery

Medicine is a broad church. In other words, once you have basic medical qualifications there are a number of career options. What you decide to do ought to be
governed by your interests, previous experience and qualifications, promotion
prospects and other personal factors.

It would be impossible in a book of this size to describe individual specialties
in detail. However, we urge you to do your own research. For example, there is
massive variation in competition for training posts in different specialties. Each
Royal College's contact details are listed at the back of the book. This could be a
starting point for your explorations. Talk to colleagues who have come to the UK
for off-the-record information about future trends, training opportunities and
other information you need to know before committing yourself. If your chosen
specialty is popular, you will have limited choices as to where you will get a job.
Be prepared to move.

■ Career paths

There are a number of possible career paths in the UK.

■ Hospital medicine

There are two distinct career pathways in hospital medicine: training-grade posts
approved for entry to membership examinations and a certificate of completion of
specialist training (CCST), and career-grade posts (*see* Figure 3.1). Recently, non-
standard hospital grades have been advertised by trusts and these are described
in greater detail later in this chapter.

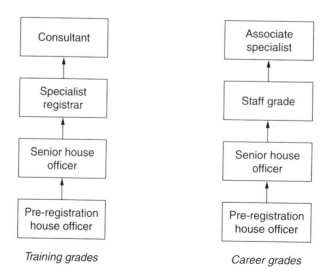

Figure 3.1 Two distinct career paths in hospital medicine.

■ General practice

GP principals (*see* Figure 3.2) are the largest group of senior doctors in the NHS. For further information *see* Chapter 4 on 'General practice'.

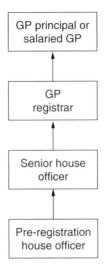

Figure 3.2 General practice career pathway.

■ Medical academia

Some doctors prefer to concentrate on research (*see* Figure 3.3). They are usually employed by universities rather than the NHS, but most hold honorary NHS contracts. Regrettably, remuneration tends to be less than their clinical counterparts, even though many have heavy clinical workloads as well.

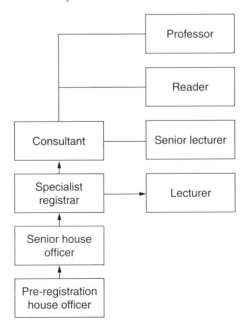

Figure 3.3 Medical academia career pathway.

■ Public health medicine (*see* Figure 3.4)

There are relatively few public health doctors. Nationwide there are hundreds rather than thousands. This specialty looks at the bigger picture: epidemiology and communicable diseases.

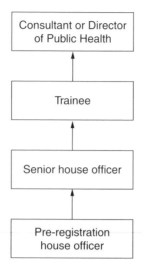

Figure 3.4 Public health career pathway.

■ Portfolio career

In a portfolio career, a doctor's working week is made up of a number of different jobs and interests.

■ **How to arrange a clinical attachment**

> If people are known to a trust through doing a clinical attachment, often the trust is then quite happy to consider them for a job in open competition. There is no old boys' network here, everything is in open competition, but if you are known it helps.
>
> Yong Lok Ong, consultant old age psychiatrist from Singapore and Overseas Doctors Dean, London Deanery

> The main advantage is that you have some understanding of the way things are done in Britain.
>
> Professor Michael Cormi, British GP

Clinical attachments are unpaid medical observer posts that give international doctors an opportunity to see how medicine is practised in the UK (*see* Box 3.1). They also provide a good opportunity to improve your medical English. Either a student visa or visitor's visa is appropriate for clinical attachments. You do not need GMC registration.

Box 3.1 Clinical attachments

On a clinical attachment you can:
- attend ward rounds
- observe in theatre
- sit in on outpatient clinics
- shadow doctors on call
- take histories and examine patients under direct supervision from a registered medical practitioner.

A clinical attachee may not:
- undertake any duties of a doctor
- work as a locum.

Arranging a clinical attachment can be very frustrating: 'I tried to get a clinical attachment and wrote to a lot of hospitals,' a refugee surgeon from the Congo who preferred to remain anonymous told us. 'None of them replied. Then by chance my son was ill and had to go to hospital. While we were in hospital with my son I met one of the consultants and asked him if I could come for a clinical attachment. He said yes.'

> When I asked my colleague how he got his attachment, he said, 'I wrote a personal letter to a named person.' I did better. I went and waited for the consultant and said, 'I would like a clinical attachment.' He said, 'Talk to my secretary, give her your CV and fill in a form.' The next day I started. Even if you arrange your own clinical attachment it might not be very organised. You can end up going round the ward on your own. If you are a shy person and not proactive it isn't going to be a good teaching experience. Some people end up doing work, which by law you are not allowed to do. If you make a mistake you are on your own.
> Otmane El Mezoued, refugee doctor from Algeria

Professor Michael Cormi is involved in a scheme funded by the North London Workforce Development Confederation for Refugee Doctors. It places refugee doctors for six weeks with a GP practice tutor and six weeks with a hospital-based tutor. He recommends doctors looking for a clinical attachment should: 'Contact the Deanery. There is an overseas doctors' dean and he should be able to facilitate clinical attachments. The main advantage of a clinical attachment is that you have some understanding of the way things are done in Britain. This may be very different from the country you come from. If you don't understand the system you won't get anywhere.'

The London Deanery organises clinical attachments for people wanting to pursue a career in general practice. Otmane El Mezoued (see above quote) did a six-week clinical attachment with a GP and found it: 'Very different from my hospital attachment. It was organised. I was taught, not exploited. There was feedback. I could ask questions about primary care and I learned a lot.'

■ Ten steps to arranging a clinical attachment

1 Prepare a winning CV (as described later in this chapter) and make sure you have documentary evidence of hepatitis B immunity.
2 Contact the postgraduate deanery and make contact with the dean responsible for overseas doctors.
3 Find out from the deanery which hospitals offer clinical attachments. Once you have a list of hospitals, the best person to approach is the clinical tutor of your chosen specialty. There will be a clinical tutor for each specialty in every trust. Alternatively, if you know any consultants, approach them directly and ask if they would be willing to have you as a clinical attachee.
4 Find out the name of the medical staffing officer for ten hospitals on your list.
5 Write a covering letter to each, stating why you want an attachment at that hospital and what you feel you can offer.
6 Mention that the clinical tutor or another consultant has indicated they would be willing for you to come.
7 Wait. While you are waiting, identify another ten hospitals that offer attachments. If you don't hear within four weeks, follow up your letter with a phone call. If you have been unsuccessful, ask why.
8 Be prepared for a lot of rejections and unanswered letters. If you are successful, the medical staffing officer will issue a letter authorising the attachment.
9 You are likely to be charged a fee. If you don't pay, you will lose your place. Some hospitals charge up to £50 per week for a clinical attachment.
10 Some hospitals will be able to offer you accommodation, but you will need to pay for it (*see* Chapter 8).

■ Training grades

> As well as Monday to Friday, nine to five, I work one of every four nights in the hospital and one in four weekends. Dread consumes the evening before the day on call as I sense impending confinement, discomfort and sleeplessness, and I consign myself to an early night. Torpor swallows the evening after the night on call. As August fades to September, I learn to cherish the one night in four I can accompany Rebecca to the cinema and not fall asleep … These things we learned the hard way.
>
> Taken from *Bodies*[1] by Jed Mercurio, doctor and writer

Recognised posts for training in the UK are as follows.

■ Pre-registration house officer (one year)

The PRHO year is undertaken by all UK doctors while provisionally registered with the GMC. PRHO posts are recognised as counting towards the pre-registration year only, not towards postgraduate training. Traditionally the PRHO year was divided into six months in medicine and six months in surgery. Recently, innovatory posts have been created offering four months in medicine, four months in surgery and four months in another specialty, including for example paediatrics, obstetrics, psychiatry and general practice.

Most PRHO posts are not advertised. This is because in most regions the postgraduate dean operates a matching scheme for final-year medical students, allocating students to PRHO posts. However, in some areas there are more PRHO posts than medical students and so some posts are advertised in the medical press. PRHO posts commence in February and August.

What does a PRHO do?

PRHOs are responsible for the day-to-day care of their team's inpatients. PRHOs administrate all new admissions. They organise investigations and carry out instructions from the consultant and other members of the multidisciplinary team. They may also assist in outpatients and theatre. Despite the New Deal (described in Chapter 2), PRHOs work long hours and this can be exhausting.

The PRHO year and non-UK medical graduates

The PRHO year is essentially the final year of UK medical training. It complements medical school education and builds on it. It is a good idea to complete pre-registration experience in your own country before coming to the UK. However, international medical graduates have benefited from working as a PRHO and found it a useful way of gaining insights into the NHS and UK medical care. If this is something you are considering, look out for adverts in the medical press and contact regional postgraduate deans.

■ Senior house officer (two to three years)

At this point doctors train in a number of different specialties and it is usual to begin to consider what eventual career path you would like to follow; for example, whether to become a GP or a hospital consultant in a specific specialty.

SHO and SpR posts (*see* below) are approved for training by the postgraduate dean and relevant Royal College. When you look at advertisements for training posts, they should contain the following statement: '*The postgraduate dean confirms that this placement and/or programme has the required educational and Dean's approval.*'

Training posts usually form part of a 'rotation' of different placements, designed to allow maximum exposure to different areas needed for membership examinations and future practice. There will be some protected time each week for formal education and also many opportunities for informal learning while you are carrying out the job. There are still a lot of so-called 'stand-alone' SHO posts which are not part of rotations. If you work in a stand-alone (non-rotating) SHO post, don't stay longer than a year otherwise your career will stand still.

Doctors can create their own SHO training package by applying every six months for jobs approved for this purpose by the relevant Royal College, but this has several disadvantages:

- There are no guarantees of securing jobs every six months.
- Periods of working as a locum in unapproved jobs may be financially lucrative but ultimately frustrating.
- Unemployment is disheartening and a source of anxiety.
- Job hunting becomes a regular chore rather than a one-off.

- Lack of continuity with doctors and other colleagues, inconsistent senior support and multiple moves around the country may have detrimental effects on interpersonal relationships and membership examination results.

■ Specialist registrar (four to five years)

This is a period of specialist training in an area that you have chosen. By the end of this stage you should have completed the relevant Royal College exams.

There are two types of SpR training:

1 *Type 1 programmes* lead to a certificate of completion of specialist training (CCST). If you are appointed to a type 1 programme, European Economic Area (EEA) nationals are given a national training number (NTN) and overseas doctors are allocated a visiting training number (VTN).
2 *Type 2 programmes* do not lead to a CCST, but are otherwise identical. If you are appointed to a type 2 programme you will be given a fixed-term training number (FTN) that is valid for the duration of your post. The duration will usually be between six and 24 months and there is usually a goal attached to the training period, such as completing an examination.

There are two types of SpR locum appointments:

1 *Locum appointment for training* (LAT) is locum cover for a doctor on a type 1 programme who is away for a fixed period, for example maternity leave. If you work in a LAT and are later appointed to a type 1 post, you can count up to 12 months of your LAT towards your CCST. Working as a LAT may help your SpR job applications, but it doesn't guarantee you an NTN or VTN.
2 *Locum appointment for service* (LAS) is locum cover in a non-training post. You cannot count it towards higher training. Doctors on permit-free training cannot work in this sort of post.

■ Staff-grade, associate specialist and trust-grade doctors

There are many doctors in a variety of non-training posts where the emphasis is on service delivery, and jobs are not part of a long-term career structure. They comprise staff grades, associate specialists, clinical assistants, hospital practitioners and non-standard, so-called 'trust' grades. Overseas doctors cannot work in these jobs on a permit-free training visa, but need a work permit.

■ Staff-grade and associate specialist doctors

Staff-grade and associate specialist doctors (SAS) have traditionally formed a large part of the medical workforce. They used to be known as non-consultant career-grade doctors and you may still see the abbreviation NCCG used. It is synonymous with SAS. There has been a rapid expansion in the number of SAS doctors since 1987. At one time there was a ceiling on the number of SAS posts. They were not to exceed 10% of the consultants in a particular specialty. Now there is no limit and trusts can appoint as many as they need.

Doctors normally take up SAS posts after working at other grades, often training grades, within their specialty. Many are tied to a locality for family reasons and others work part time. SAS doctors are a heterogenous group with different needs. Clinical teams with heavy service pressures often leave SAS doctors with massive clinical workloads and limited educational opportunities. Boxes 3.2 and 3.3 list some advantages and disadvantages of SAS posts.

Box 3.2 Advantages of SAS posts

- A secure career
- No need to take professional exams (although many do)
- No overall 24-hour responsibility for patients
- No antisocial hours or on-call
- Increased opportunities for part-time working
- No need to move around the country on rotations

Box 3.3 Disadvantages of SAS posts

- Poor career advice before entry
- Variable work content which may be at an inappropriately high or low level
- Variable supervision
- Poor educational opportunities
- Limited or no opportunities for career progression. In order to become a consultant, SAS doctors need to apply for an NTN and higher specialist training in open competition

---

Dr Nat Lawson was the first staff-grade physician in South-East England. He works in care of elderly medicine at Pembury Hospital, Tunbridge Wells. He is often overworked due to staff shortages: 'There are three staff-grade doctors here. There ought to be four but they can't get a fourth person.' His clinical role is not clearly defined and has expanded over his decade in the post: 'I do the work of a whole team: house officer, SHO, specialist registrar. I do all of it. In the clinic, because they haven't replaced the consultant, I see the new patients he would have seen. I've agreed to do that and I'm not complaining. But that wasn't the agreement initially.'

The New Deal has been a bad deal for Nat: 'The SHOs all get protected sleep, but there are no bleep-free periods for me. When the SHOs were overworked, people helped to reduce their workload, but I've ended up doing their work on top of my other work.' Nat also lacks protected time for continuing professional development (CPD): 'I try to go to meetings to stay up to date when I can, but it is difficult for them to find locums when I go off,' he says. 'I have never had any study leave because nobody would cover my ward work. I used to go to regular hypertension updates, but I don't feel comfortable leaving the ward without someone to cover me.'

Nat believes staff-grade doctors offer patients more: 'Staff-grade doctors are more devoted to patients than other doctors as we are not always moving here and there and worrying about going home at five o'clock. We do as much as possible and we stay late to get it all done. Most other doctors would be off home, but we are more committed.'

Dr Susanna Swallow is a staff grade in clinical haematology at Rotherham General Hospital. Her job was converted from clinical assistant to staff grade two years ago. She works four and a half sessions per week and describes her job as 'fitting in well with family commitments'. Her consultants have encouraged CPD and she is pleased to have accrued 'all my CPD points for the Royal College of Pathologists folder'.

Susanna feels she is doing one doctor's work rather than a whole team's and says, 'There is consultant support available 99.99% of the time. It is unusual for there not to be either a consultant there or one on the end of a phone.'

She explains several advantages available to her as an SAS doctor: 'I get to do clinical work which I enjoy, but I don't have to fight my corner or get involved with a lot of politics.' But she recognises that it might not be for everyone: 'I wouldn't do a staff-grade job if I wanted to be a consultant. It wouldn't suit a person who wants to be in charge. I'm happy not to be King Pin.'

Dr Korangatnu Valsraj is a specialist registrar in psychiatry at the Maudsley Hospital, London. After finishing an SHO rotation, he worked as a staff-grade psychiatrist, working with the Home Treatment Team in South London and Maudsley NHS Trust. Like many international doctors, he found himself with no option but to take a staff-grade job. He explains: 'Home Office regulations are very strict and they only allow overseas doctors to work as an SHO for four years. My visa could not be extended unless the postgraduate dean approved. Despite support from many consultants, the clinical tutor, medical director and director of postgraduate education, bureaucracy worked against me and I was forced to become a staff-grade doctor.'

Like Susanna, Korangatnu found some aspects of the staff-grade role advantageous: 'I enjoyed the clinical work; I worked with an excellent team in an innovative area and learned a lot about setting up a new service from scratch in line with the National Service Framework. I wouldn't have got that out of an SHO job because the job wasn't approved by the Royal College for SHO training.' He may have hit the concrete ceiling but was helped out and up. As soon as he passed his membership exams he moved on to higher specialist training.

The BMA has a separate committee for SAS doctors, which aims to address poor pay, training and career progression and promotes the SAS doctors' contribution to the NHS. The chairman, Dr Mohib Khan, holds strong views on the future for SAS doctors. He can be contacted through the BMA.

■ Trust-grade doctors

> Lots of people are clutching at straws for survival and go into trust-grade jobs, finding that they are dead-end jobs.
>
> Yong Lok Ong, consultant old age psychiatrist from Singapore and Overseas Doctors Dean, London Deanery

> Forget about trust posts. Think very hard. You had better know what you are getting into.
>
> Anuga Shedeo, PLAB candidate from India

Trust-grade posts are in fact non-standard, non-training grade posts. These posts are advertised with titles that do not conform to nationally recognised hospital grades, and include:

- admissions ward officer
- clinical research associate
- junior clinical fellow, SHO equivalent
- locum trust house officer
- non-heart-beating kidney-donor transplantation fellow.

Trusts are inventive and there are far too many job titles to be listed here. As a rule of thumb, any post which does not conform to one of the job titles below (training and career grades) is a trust-grade post.

Training grades
house officer
senior house officer
specialist registrar
senior registrar

Career grades
staff grade
associate specialist
clinical assistant
hospital practitioner

BMA advice is that junior hospital posts should 'contain prominently the statement: "The postgraduate dean confirms that this placement and/or programme has the educational and dean's approval."' There is a surprisingly high proportion of non-standard grade jobs advertised in the UK throughout the year.[2] Doctors employed on local terms and conditions of service are becoming a major source of service delivery as trusts struggle to meet service requirements while implementing the New Deal's requirements.

These doctors, typically from non-EEA countries, may be misled by ambiguous job titles and, unlike their training-grade colleagues, they are not entitled to educational supervision. Don't be misled by job titles claiming to be 'SHO equivalent'. The workload may well be equivalent but there is no guarantee that you will have the same educational opportunites as SHOs. Furthermore, any time spent in these posts, which are not approved by the postgraduate dean, will not count towards membership exams or basic specialist training.

At the time of writing, the Department of Health has published a consultation document, *Choice and Opportunity*, reviewing the difficulties and problems which occur in SAS posts. It can be accessed on www.doh.gov.uk/modernising medicalcareers/.

■ Resident medical officers in the private sector

There are approximately 230 private hospitals in the UK. Most have a resident medical officer (RMO) on site 24 hours a day, seven days a week. RMOs cover private hospitals for emergencies and general ward work; some hospitals may require them to assist in theatre. An RMO post may be less demanding than many NHS posts.

RMO work may be a good opportunity for international doctors who need to study and earn a good salary. Private hospitals vary in size, complexity of cases and workload. Many private hospitals deal exclusively with elective surgery. Private hospitals generally do not accept patients requiring acute medical admissions. Only larger private hospitals have intensive care units. This means an RMO's clinical work consists mainly of ward work and managing postoperative complications.

■ Essential experience for an RMO post

This includes:

- 12 months' clinical experience as a qualified doctor
- plus at least six months' post-registration experience (SHO equivalent) in one or more of the following:
  - medicine
  - emergency medicine
  - intensive therapy unit (ITU)
  - paediatrics
  - anaesthetics
- you must be able to lead cardiopulmonary resuscitation (CPR)
- ability to deal safely with emergencies until a consultant arrives
- in addition to your medical degree you need an advanced certificate in life support (ACLS), medical defence cover, full GMC registration, and a work permit or Grandparent Entry Certificate.

RMO jobs can be a way into working in the UK and RMOs can apply for other NHS posts while earning approximately £1500 per week, with additional holiday pay. RMOs usually work 168-hour shifts and need to remain on site for the whole span of duty. Outside of normal working hours (9am to 5pm), the RMO is the only doctor on site. If you are considering working as an RMO, you must be competent and confident in dealing with clinical emergencies, including cardiac arrests. Meals and accommodation are free whilst on duty and the on-call room will usually have satellite TV.

Typically RMOs work for one week, then have the next week off. However, they may work for two weeks and then only have one week off. Most private hospitals provide accommodation to RMOs during duty weeks only. Some may allow you to leave luggage in a safe place while you are off duty, but you probably will need somewhere else to live when you are not working. You might be able to pair up with another RMO and share rent on your other accommodation.

■ Locums

> I locumed for a couple of months and then went travelling for a month, then came back and locumed for some more money. That was fun. I joined locum agencies and thought psychiatry would be interesting to do, and it was. I did it to supplement my travel around Europe. I went to Germany, France, Italy, Morocco and Turkey in between locum jobs. I was never money greedy. I never felt exploited and had a good time.
>
> Stephanie Young, SpR psychiatrist from New Zealand

> Locums are exploited by substantive doctors, employers, agencies, in short everyone. Locums are discriminated against in every aspect of the profession. Their contract, rights, entitlements and benefits are less than those of substantive doctors. They are excluded from many areas of decision-making within hospital departments.
>
> Shehnaz Somjee, Founding Chairperson of the
> Locum Doctors Association

> I came to Bury as a locum for eight days because somebody fell ill. I stayed for four years. At the end of the eight-day locum, I became an SHO and then a registrar. Later a consultant job came up at Bury where I had been a junior doctor for four years. And I got it.
>
> Umesh Prabhu, consultant paediatrician from India

Locums are an essential part of the NHS workforce. Locums are used because posts are vacant or because permanent staff are on leave. Placements vary from weekend and evening work to long contracts and permanent placements. You can give your details to a locum agency, who advertise in the medical press. This is the most common route for hospital locums, but less common for GP locums.

■ GP locums

GP locums should send their CV and a covering letter to practices they want to work for. In many areas there are non-principal groups that distribute locum lists to the practices in their locality. There is often a fee of £10–£20 per year for this.

■ Advantages of locum work

Advantages include:

- you choose where and when you work
- experience of different teams and trusts
- you develop a portfolio of skills and contacts
- highly paid work.

■ Agencies

Agencies make money by charging the hospital more than your hourly rate and keeping the difference, so remember they work for you. Some agencies specialise in short-term work which is ideal if you are looking to work in the evenings or weekends. Others offer longer term placements. Certain agencies have special expertise in helping overseas doctors with visas. Large agencies tend to pay higher rates (*see* Box 3.4), but work offers are more infrequent. Smaller agencies may pay less but often contact you more frequently. You need to be contacted easily or the agency will go elsewhere, as it is usually 'first come, first served'. If you are prepared to travel you will have a greater choice of jobs, but negotiate travel expenses and make sure you get good accommodation.

Box 3.4 Typical hourly locum rates

Pre-registration house officer – £22.50
Senior house officer – £30
Specialist registrar – £40
Staff grade – £45
Consultant – £85

■ Registering with an agency

Register with no more than three locum agencies. Be very specific about what kinds of jobs you would like in terms of location and hours, and don't be coerced into doing extra hours. If the job they give you is hideous, don't feel you have to stay. You are your own boss. Don't compromise yourself in any way and don't feel you have to do jobs in the back of nowhere.

Stephanie Young, SpR psychiatrist from New Zealand

We suggest you contact several agencies and get answers to the following:

- How much of the sort of work you are looking for do they have in your specialty?
- What is the hourly rate?
- Is there a higher rate at nights and weekends?

- Is there holiday pay? You should get this.
- Are there any incentives? Some offer money if you recommend a friend.
- Do they have an online database of available jobs and how often is it updated?
- Can you book jobs online?

To work out which agencies to join, ask at the hospital where you want to work. Ask medical staffing officers or locums working at the hospital which agencies they use.

■ European Working Time Directive

Remember that the European Working Time Directive still applies (*see* p. 22). If you work as a locum while in a substantive post you will be breaking the law if you do work in excess of the EWTD. Many doctors get round this by doing some extra on-call duties during their annual leave.

■ Training

One of the drawbacks of working as a locum is that opportunities for formal, recognised training are drastically reduced.

> Being a 'locum' in itself serves to disqualify a doctor from training, public appointments and research grants, and prejudices the CV as being a 'rolling stone gathering no moss'. Our employers think that a locum CV is less competitive than a substantive CV simply because of the short duration of posts. They ignore the skills and experience locums do pick up. The only recognised training locum posts are LATS SpRs. These are very few and far between. It is currently extremely difficult to get any training in locum posts because locums are not seen or recognised as trainees. Locums are, however, able to pick up much in posts through their own initiative, with little or no thanks to their employers, most of whom actively discourage locums to participate in learning. This indicates most locums are keen and quick to teach and train.
>
> Shehnaz Somjee

■ The Locum Doctors Association

The Locum Doctors Association (LDA) is the only trade union of locum doctors. It negotiates on behalf of locums. The LDA offers free membership to unemployed and refugee doctors. Its services include dispute resolution with employers and agencies and legal, medico-legal and career-related advice and assistance. It also provides assistance with GMC matters. The LDA has seats on government and professional bodies and is able to influence change.

> Many locums do not join until after they have problems. We stress that our membership is like an insurance policy. If you are insured you have

no worries and we are there for you when you need us. We can also help prevent problems, some of which are incurable or difficult to resolve.

Shehnaz Somjee, Founding Chairperson of the
Locum Doctors Association

■ Finding a job

I left India because I was not progressing because of my caste. I did my PLAB examination and applied for 72 jobs and was not shortlisted for any, despite my distinctions and Diploma in Child Health.

Umesh Prabhu, consultant paediatrician from India

People say you can't get a job, but I had two interviews on the same day and I was offered both jobs in the teaching hospital. I was a bit shocked.

Arshana Mishra, SHO in paediatrics from India

Getting your dream job is a four-stage process:

1 job hunting
2 dispatching a tailor-made CV/application form
3 interview preparation
4 interview.

PRHO jobs tend to be arranged by medical schools for UK graduates. A minority are advertised. Almost all other jobs (SHO, SpR, associate specialists, staff grade, non-standard grade jobs, locum work and consultant posts) are advertised in *BMJ Careers*, a supplement of the *British Medical Journal* (*BMJ*). This is available online and you can sign up to receive free email alerts of jobs that match your requirements.

Jobs are also advertised in:

• *Hospital Doctor* – a free weekly newspaper that you may find in medical libraries and lying around in the doctors' mess
• the *Lancet* – you should be able to find a copy in most medical libraries.

However, it should be noted that most academic posts are not formally advertised.

Make a list of what you want from a job. You might like to consider the balance between service and training and the importance of a social life. Do you want to live in a city or the countryside? Are there suitable schools nearby? Does the job fit in with your lifestyle? Compile a list of posts matching most of your expectations.

The advertisement will usually only provide minimal details about the job. It will also contain instructions on how to apply. This may be by CV or a particular application form. Follow these instructions to the letter. Don't send in a CV if they have not asked for one. It will go in the bin.

Before you apply for the job, phone and ask for a 'person specification'. This sets out the desirable and essential characteristics and qualifications needed (*see* Box 3.5). You need to scrutinise this and tailor your application accordingly.

Box 3.5 Example person specification

	Essential criteria	Desirable criteria
Qualifications	MBBS or equivalent	BSc/BA (Hons)
Experience	Satisfactory completion of PRHO posts or equivalent.	Time spent in specialty on a medical student elective or a special study module. Post-qualification experience in specialty.
Knowledge		Distinction or prizes in specialty at medical school.
Clinical skills	Competent in basic procedures, e.g. history taking, physical examination, basic investigation interpretation and basic life support.	
Research	Understanding principles of research.	Experience of presenting data. Has participated in research. Peer-reviewed publication.
Audit	Understanding of audit principles.	Completed audit cycle.
Teaching	Able to contribute to clinical teaching.	Additional teaching experience.
Management	Able to prioritise clinical need.	Uses initiative.
Other	GMC registration (full or limited). Hepatitis B immunity. Satisfactory enhanced disclosure.	Driving licence.

Consultants and medical staffing officers will compile a list of suitable applicants. The more closely your CV or application form matches the person specification, the more likely you are to be put on this list, known as the shortlist. If you are shortlisted, you will be called for an interview. Successful candidates are offered jobs. If you accept a job offer, this is a legally binding agreement.

■ CVs and application forms

I have never had to fill in an application form or write a CV in my life. You hear about people making 500 applications and not being shortlisted. What are the criteria for being shortlisted?

Anuga Shedeo, PLAB candidate from India

Unless you can write a suitable CV, you won't get anywhere.

Professor Michael Cormi, British GP

Your curriculum vitae (CV) is your first and perhaps only marketing tool. It is easy to become blinkered by a desire to compose an academically accurate and impressive document that leaves no space to showcase other qualities. If you have talents that would benefit the hospital, colleagues or patients, these should be highlighted. Use no more than two sides of A4, a standard font and good-quality paper.

■ A model CV

- Full name and qualifications
- Date of birth
- Home address
- Contact phone number and email
- GMC registration details: number and type of registration
- Home office details, e.g. permit-free training, EEA national, refugee
- University and medical school
- Prizes and distinctions
- Date of primary medical qualification
- Postgraduate medical qualifications:
  - dates and awarding bodies.
- Employment to date:
  - list all your jobs in chronological order. Give UK equivalents of job titles.
- Include details of clinical attachments here
- Experience:
  - write a short paragraph summarising experience and skills gained in the posts above
  - focus on clinical skills, teaching and management experience as well as specific experience in the UK.
- Courses:
  - list all relevant courses attended, for example ACLS or medical ethics, in chronological order. Don't include exam-oriented revision courses for exams you have since passed.
- Research:
  - briefly outline research you have been involved in and state the extent of your involvement. List papers published in chronological order and give full references. Don't make anything up.
- Audit:
  - summarise all audit projects you have been involved in and state what the outcome was. What did you find? Was the audit loop closed?

- Teaching:
  - list presentations or lectures you have given, including informal teaching of junior doctors, medical students and nurses. Also mention any non-medical teaching that you have provided.
- Positions of responsibility:
  - include tasks such as organising on-call rotas, committee membership and doctors' representative. State your achievements in post.
- Outside interests:
  - include things you are genuinely interested in and can talk about. Don't include things you have only done once or twice. It will reflect badly on you at interview if you are asked about them.
- Referees:
  - ask referees for permission before you use them. Tell them about your application and ask for their support. Give them a copy of your CV. Check you have spelled their names correctly.

■ Adapt your CV

You may need several slightly different CVs depending on the post. Human resources (HR) usually send an application pack with a list of essential and desirable characteristics. Write your CV, highlighting desirable characteristics with supportive examples. For instance, if 'organised' is cited as a desirable quality, an applicant might write: 'I am organised and efficient, key skills I used in my role as cricket club captain when I assumed responsibility for organising the team's activities.'

Job advertisements will state the number of copies required, and it would be foolish not to be shortlisted because this simple specification was overlooked. Retain a copy, especially when using different formats for different rotations.

■ Application forms

If you are required to complete an application form instead of sending your CV, don't send a CV. It will end up in the bin. Use your CV to fill in the application form, ensuring you don't leave any sections blank. Answer the form in as much detail as possible. Write neatly or type answers into the space provided. Don't use any extra paper. It is a good idea to photocopy the application form and use the spare to plan your answers. Discuss them with a senior colleague first.

■ Interviews

When I came here I went for an interview. It was a disaster. I had no idea about what an interview is, or about how to prepare for it. Back home we don't have job interviews. If you want a job someone will recommend you. The panel must have been shocked by the way I answered questions. I felt really bad. They didn't test knowledge, they wanted to see how I coped under pressure. They asked me about personal experiences and I wasn't expecting that. I was asked to give examples of how I had done things.

Otmane El Mezoued, refugee doctor from Algeria

■ Interview preparation

Once you have an interview date, speak to some key players such as the following:

- *a doctor in post.* A doctor in post may be the best person to tell you what the job is really like and how it differs from the job advert. This doctor should also be able to give you honest answers about accommodation, senior support and practical advice such as availability of food out-of-hours. Perhaps on paper you work a half-day after an on-call, but your informant may advise you that this rarely happens due to other commitments like an outpatient clinic.
- *human resources/medical staffing.* The human resources department or its medical staffing subdivision will be able to answer questions about leave allowances, locum cover and pay banding for all jobs. Many are willing to send out a sample contract. There is nothing to stop you from sending this to your local BMA office to ensure it is legally sound.

If your CV or application form is your entry ticket, then the interview is your chance to shine. Think positively. If you were not considered a suitable candidate for the job, you would not have made the shortlist.

■ What to wear

First impressions count. Dressing appropriately for a job interview is critical. The message you want to convey to your prospective employers is that you are a trustworthy and knowledgeable professional. The correct attire encourages interview panels to take you and what you say seriously. Your clothes should be smarter than what you would wear for work. Clothing should always be impeccably clean, crisp, pressed and in good condition. Shoes should shine.

Don't wear:

- heavy or jangling jewellery
- loud colours
- excessively patterned clothes
- anything revealing or uncomfortable.

Be remembered for what you said, not for how you looked.

■ The interview itself

Aim to get there half an hour early and add extra time for complicated journeys. Use this time to have a final look over your CV and application form. Read a serious newspaper. Many interviewers try to put you at ease by making some opening small talk about topical events. When you meet an interview panel, try to remember their names and make good eye contact. A warm smile, confident handshake and positive presence are invaluable. Psychologists have found most of us decide what someone else is like within the first few seconds of meeting them. There is no reason why interviewers should not conform.

Interviews are a two-way process. It is worth remembering that you are also interviewing the panel. Instead of wondering nervously if they are impressed by your responses, ask yourself if you want to work in this trust with these people.

At the end of the interview, it is customary for panels to ask candidates if they have any questions. This is another opportunity to excel. Most questions merely demonstrate a lack of homework, leaving a poor impression. Much better is a rejoiner such as: 'I've already spoken to the postgraduate dean, Dr Brown, currently on your rotation, and also the human resources department, and between them they have answered all my questions.'

Tips for good interview technique

- Be prepared for questions. Before the interview consider what you could be asked and prepare. When you are asked a question, you will already have an answer that can be adapted.
- Ask a colleague or friend to interview you and rehearse how you will answer. You will brush up on skills and appear more confident on the day.
- Take a deep breath and try to relax as you go into the interview room.
- Smile, make eye contact with the interviewers as you are introduced to them and shake their hands. A friendly approach will make you look upbeat and interesting.
- Think about your answers before starting to speak.
- Try to be confident and positive when answering.
- If you are asked a question that you don't understand, ask the panel to explain it. This is better than answering the wrong question and shows you are not afraid to ask for help when needed.
- Making a mistake during an interview is not the end of the world.
- Highlight achievements and accomplishments.
- Never lie about qualifications that you do not have. You will be found out and this will ruin employment prospects.

If you are not appointed after being interviewed it might be due to:

- too many other applicants meeting essential and desirable criteria
- poor personal appearance
- inability to express ideas and opinions clearly
- lack of confidence
- overconfidence
- poor references.

■ How to get a specialist registrar training post

After getting an SHO post you realise that is the least of your struggles. The main bottleneck is getting SpR posts.

Samja Mishra, SHO in ophthalmology from India

Specialist registrar interviews are tough. In some specialties there are more than a dozen talented and highly motivated candidates for each training post. This section highlights some issues you might have to address and offers suggestions that might help you answer various questions.

'*Do you have gaps in your CV?*' If your CV was complete you would be applying to head an internationally renowned department. Emphasise achievements so far, for instance passing your membership exams first time, together with experiences you would like to have had, given unlimited time as an SHO. Explain exactly how you aim to make up for these shortcomings as soon as you are on the SpR rotation. You might say something like: 'I don't have any peer-reviewed publications, but during my informal visit I discussed my research interests with Professor Green and he has kindly agreed to be my research supervisor if I am appointed.' Or tell them about the case series you have pending. This may precipitate a question about your research interests. You can also use this question to demonstrate where you have gone the extra mile to gain experience not readily available to you. For instance, 'Although I haven't got the Diploma in Child Health, I arranged to sit in on paediatric outpatients and found this useful.' Don't finish answering this question without adding a sentence about why you now feel ready to move to the SpR grade.

'*Tell me about a memorable case where you learned something new.*' This might also be phrased as '*What's the worst case you have managed?*' or '*What's the most interesting case you have seen?*' It is important to remember that these are essentially the same question in different guises. Don't talk about a near miss, even if it has a happy ending. You need to be seen as a competent, conscientious and confident doctor, not a lucky chancer. Give a succinct account of the patient. Outline the difficulty. Explain how it was overcome. The case you prepare in advance to answer this question should demonstrate your willingness to learn from more senior colleagues, and your ability to reason scientifically, apply literature appropriately and reflect productively on a changing clinical picture. Give the panel examples of how your involvement in that case has changed the way you work.

'*What are your career intentions?*' It is highly likely that you will be asked about your future aspirations. You may also be asked '*What are your aims and objectives for your time on the SpR rotation?*', which needs to be answered in the light of another favourite, '*Where do you see yourself in five years' time?*' You need to decide what sort of consultant you want to be. Do you want to work in a district general hospital, teaching hospital or do you want to be an academic? Tell the panel about a consultant who has particularly impressed you and what qualities you consider to be essential. Explain how you will acquire or hone these characteristics yourself on their rotation. You need to be familiar with what is on offer and have contacted key players prior to the interview.

'*What do you understand by audit?*' Take a deep breath before trotting out: 'By the process of audit a potentially modifiable treatment or process is assessed and compared to a standard. Shortfalls are identified and rectified and then the process is repeated.' Illustrate your answer with practical examples from previous experience. Even if you have got this far without undertaking an audit yourself, it adds authenticity to talk about an audit undertaken in your department. Alternatively, you may be invited to *'Describe your audit experience'*. Before launching into an explanation of a half-completed audit cycle you were coerced into three years ago, set the scene. Summarise current audit projects your department is involved in, highlight any personal involvement and say why it is important to you. If you have done an audit, explain the background, process and outcomes. Tell them whether the audit loop was closed. SHOs often leave audits mid-cycle as they move jobs. Mentioning it demonstrates that you know it is important, and tell the panel who will be closing the audit loop on your behalf.

'What are your research interests?' You need to be able to talk about an important area or recent paper. If you don't have one, revise a topic you are fluent and familiar with. It helps to know about a recent paper from a specialist journal, so that you are equally equipped to answer *'Tell me about a recent paper that has changed your practice'*. Don't gush about your interviewers' research interests unless you genuinely share them. If you are asked *'Should every trainee undertake research?'*, say yes, as involvement in research gives trainees skills and under-standing of methodology, design, statistics and data analysis. Lots of aspiring SpRs feel strongly that they shouldn't have to do excessive research just to get shortlisted. The interview isn't the forum for that debate.

'What do you understand by clinical governance?' Clinical governance is the means by which health organisations meet their duty of quality assurance at local level. NHS organisations are accountable for continuously improving their services and ensuring high standards of care. Remember the components of clinical governance using the mnemonic QC Read:

- **Q**uality improvement
- **C**ontinuing professional development
- **R**isk reduction
- **E**vidence-based medicine
- **A**udit
- **D**evelopment of information strategies.

Be prepared to talk about any aspect in more detail.

'What do you think about nurse prescribing?' and *'Why do we need evidence when we have opinion?'* are just two examples of thorny topics where there is no correct answer. If you have an answer ready you can demonstrate deft diplomatic and political skills, much valued at SpR level. You need to memorise a brief list of arguments for and against each position. Editorials in specialist journals are a good source. A suggested framework for answering thorny questions is:

This is a contentious issue …
On one hand …
On the other hand …
On balance, my own view is …

The selection high bar is raised every year. At SpR level, everyone shortlisted is highly qualified and comes highly recommended. Clinical excellence is not enough.

Awareness of health service politics, clinical governance and your specialty's hot topics are imperative.

■ References

1 Mercurio J (2003) *Bodies*. Vintage, London.

2 Dosani S, Schroter S, MacDonald R *et al.* (2003) Recruitment of doctors to non-standard grades in the NHS: analysis of job advertisements and survey of advertisers. *BMJ*. **327**: 961–4.

■ Further reading

BMJ Careers devoted a theme issue to trust-grade doctors: *BMJ Careers*, 25 October 2003.

Constantine S and Woodall T (2003) *What Not to Wear 2: for every occasion*. Weidenfield Nicolson, London.

Flusser A (2003) *Dressing the Man*. HarperCollins, London.

Houston K (1998) *Creating Winning CVs and Applications*. Trotman, Richmond, Surrey.

Turya E (2003) *Your Career After PLAB: survival tools for young doctors*. Edukom, Manchester.

Ward C and Eccles S (2001) *So You Want To Be A Brain Surgeon?* Oxford University Press, Oxford.

CHAPTER 4

General practice

We have devoted a chapter to general practice to reflect its importance to the NHS and also the career opportunities for international doctors wishing to work in the UK.

Everyone living in the UK is entitled to register with a general practitioner (GP). There are approximately 31 000 GPs working here,[1] providing an impressive and comprehensive network of healthcare and support. While it is true that patients do get admitted to hospital from accident and emergency (A&E) departments, the vast majority are referred by their GP, sometimes known as the 'family doctor'.

But hospital referrals are only the tip of the iceberg. Many more patients are seen and treated either directly by their GP or by other colleagues working in primary care. The variety of patients, conditions and treatments undertaken by GPs is staggering. Good GPs, of which there are many, need to be able to see, assess, diagnose, consider further investigations, prescribe treatments or make referrals in seven minutes. They are often the first point of contact for patients who arrive with new presentations, and they see each patient on their list on average four or five times each year.

Despite the demands placed on GPs and the increasing expectations of patients, the primary care system works well and GPs are frequently polled as the most trusted and respected professionals in British society.

■ Why consider general practice?

- Ample opportunities for international doctors.
- Scope to practise anywhere in the UK.
- Varied and interesting clinical work.
- GPs treat patients from 'cradle to grave'.
- Potential to develop autonomy and entrepreunership as well as undertaking sessional work.
- Unique experiences at the front line of medical care.
- Chance to be part of a dynamic specialty with increasing research opportunities.
- Ideal career for team players.
- Clinical work uses a holistic model of healthcare.
- Opportunities to develop a special interest.

■ Recruitment crisis

Another good reason for considering a career in general practice is the national recruitment crisis. Yvonne Carter, a professor of general practice and primary care at St Bartholomew's (Barts) and the London Queen Mary School of Medicine and Dentistry, has called it 'a national time bomb'.[2]

A generation of international doctors, especially from the commonwealth countries (in particular India and Sri Lanka), who took up GP posts in the 1960s and 1970s are coming up to retirement age and there are insufficient newly qualified doctors to replace them. The increasing number of women doctors means that there are more doctors going into general practice who wish to work part time as a 'salaried GP' rather than as a practice partner and so-called 'principal'. Recruitment is especially difficult in certain deprived areas and inner-city practices.

As a result, 'golden hello' schemes have been instigated by the Government. Currently, new GP recruits are being offered £6000 upon appointment to a GP post, with an additional £6000 for those working in deprived areas such as the former industrial areas in South Wales and the North-East of England.

> Almost from the moment I knew I wanted to be a doctor, I wanted to be a GP. The reason is I like people, I like working with families, and what I like most about it is that you see the same people over and over again. I've never been so keen on the sort of medicine where you see somebody and do a hip replacement and that's the last time you ever see them. That's not for me. What I like is the longitudinal look of people. You look at their family, you look at them over a period of years, you know their husbands and their kids and their cousins, and get a real feel for that person. That has always attracted me to it. So general practice is what I've wanted to do. It's not something I drifted into, I always actively wanted to be a GP.
>
> Howard Stoate, GP and Member of Parliament

> I've been in general practice for 30 years and I would say it's a fantastic job. There are very few jobs in medicine as exciting and interesting as general practice. It's being a detective – you never know who is going to walk through the door, you never know how far it will stretch your knowledge and capability – and some of us find that exciting and interesting.
>
> Professor Michael Cormi, British GP

> During the 15 years I've been a GP, I've built a new surgery and a healthy-living centre. That sort of option is just not available in hospital. I'm seeing people now I delivered as babies. The relationship you have with them is fantastic, and outside their families there are very few relationships like that.
>
> Sam Everington, GP principal and barrister

■ Routes into UK general practice

The Joint Committee on Postgraduate Training for General Practice (JCPTGP) licenses doctors to work in UK general practice. To work as a UK GP you need to have either a JCPTGP Certificate of Prescribed Experience or a JCPTGP Certificate of Equivalent Experience, or acquired rights.

■ JCPTGP Certificate of Prescribed Experience

To obtain a JCPTGP Certificate of Prescribed Experience doctors need to spend three years in training. This is known as a vocational training scheme (VTS) and consists of:
- 12 months in approved SHO hospital posts, which might include:
  - not less than six months or more than 12 months in two of: general medicine, geriatric medicine, paediatrics or psychiatry
  - or not less than six months or more than 12 months in A&E or general surgery or A&E and orthopaedic surgery
  - or not less than six months or more than 12 months in obstetrics and gynaecology or obstetrics or gynaecology
- 12 months as a registrar in general practice or part-time pro rata equivalent and passing summative assessment
- 12 months in other approved posts, usually based in hospital.

Vocational training schemes are evolving with a move to include more community-based posts – for example, community paediatrics, community obstetrics and community psychiatry – to make them more relevant to general practice.

■ Visa regulations

It is possible to undertake the hospital SHO posts with limited GMC registration and permit-free training. However, full GMC registration is needed for the GP registrar year.

■ EEA doctors

Doctors from the EEA who have certificates of specific training or acquired rights do not need a JCPTGP certificate to work in UK general practice. It is often possible to work as a GP registrar to become more familiar with general practice in the UK.

■ Acquired rights

Doctors with a primary medical qualification from an EEA country other than the UK, who were working as doctors with full GMC registration in the UK on 31 December 1994, may practise in the UK without undertaking vocational training. The European Directive 1993/16/EEC has caused problems for some EEA doctors who graduated before 1995. Some have not been allowed to take up GP registrar posts after completing the hospital component of the VTS. We advise doctors in this position to contact the JCPTGP for advice.

■ JCPTGP Certificate of Equivalent Experience

The JCPTGP assesses international doctors' training according to UK regulations. General practice does not exist in everyone's country of graduation or may be very different. If doctors have not worked as GPs in the UK before they make recommendations for further training, ranging from a minimum of three months as a GP registrar to a full three-year VTS.

Examples

1 Mark Dawson is a 42-year-old experienced GP from New Zealand. He has an excellent CV and three good references.
   JCPTGP recommendation: three months as a GP registrar plus some aspects, but not all, of the summative assessment.

2 Faisal Ali is a 31-year-old family doctor. He has been working in a private hospital in Saudi Arabia, predominantly in obstetrics and gynaecology, for the past three years.
   JCPTGP recommendation: Dr Ali has been working in a specialist area, rather than an equivalent to UK general practice. Depending on his other postgraduate experience, the JCPTGP would recommend a minimum of three months as a GP registrar plus a maximum of three years in a VTS. JCPTGP recommendations depend on the experience doctors have.

3 John Morgan is a 29-year-old hospital doctor from Cape Town, South Africa. He has worked in a number of different specialties: paediatrics, emergency medicine, old age medicine, gynaecology and liaison psychiatry.
   JCPTGP recommendation: this doctor may be in a similar position to UK doctors who have worked in several different areas as an SHO. The JCPTGP would ask him to document what he has been doing and assess it. He may have done the equivalent of the UK VTS, but if he has been working as a medical officer rather than in a training post, the JCPTGP wouldn't consider that to be equivalent to a UK training-approved SHO post.

■ Summative assessment

Summative assessment is a test of minimum competence required of all GP registrars. Satisfactory completion of summative assessment is required in order to fill any medical role in general practice other than that of a GP registrar.

Key areas tested by summative assessment
- Knowledge
- Problem-solving skills
- Clinical competence
- Consulting/communication skills
- Skills in producing a written piece of work on general practice
- A wide variety of skills, attitudes and knowledge, confirmed by a trainer's report.

The components of summative assessment
- A test of knowledge by multiple-choice questions (MCQ)
- An assessment of consultation skills
- A written submission of practical work
- Structured trainers' report.

■ General practitioners with a special interest (GPwSI)

Although generalists by definition, some GPs choose to specialise in an area that particularly interests them. A GPwSI is a GP with appropriate experience who can deliver specialist services independently, usually outside the scope of primary care.

As well as providing variety and increased job satisfaction for individual practitioners, GPwSI reduce hospital waiting times, offer a more convenient service to patients and reduce pressures on consultants in secondary care.

Areas in which GPs commonly specialise include:

- family planning
- substance misuse
- mental health
- paediatrics.

■ Types of practice

GPs work in different types of practices: single-handed, group practices or health centres. These are found in a variety of settings: rural, urban and inner-city.

■ Single-handed practice

A single-handed practice is staffed by a lone GP, who usually employs other primary care staff such as a practice nurse and receptionist. Single-handed practices are becoming less common. Plus points include autonomy, little need for compromise with colleagues and relative freedom from bureaucracy. However, this must be weighed against the risks of professional isolation and burnout, particularly in geographically remote areas.

■ Group practice

A group practice is made up of two or more GPs in partnership. The advantages include mutual support, a chance to share and discuss complex cases, scope to develop special interests and the sharing of expertise. Partners in a group practice may own the building from which they work.

■ Health centre

Health centres are run by local trusts. They are a base for GPs and also for many other members of the primary care team. The emphasis is on teamwork.

■ Rural practice

A rural practice may be the only medical facility in a remote area. GPs need good acute medical skills. The advantages are a fairly fixed population who the GP will get to know well, often stunning surroundings, larger and more affordable housing than in the inner city, and many opportunities for outdoors activities. However, it can be difficult to have a private life as rural GPs are often high-profile members of their local communities.

■ Urban practice

These tend to be in less beautiful surroundings than rural practices, but are usually closer to hospitals. GPs in urban practices usually have a very mixed patient list, ranging from unemployed single mothers to affluent professional families. Urban practices tend to be group rather than single-handed practices. It is easier for GPs to have a private life and a degree of anonymity outside work, especially if they live in a different area from their practice.

■ Inner-city practice

Practices in the inner city offer primary healthcare to people from very deprived backgrounds. Poverty, poor housing, overcrowding, high levels of morbidity, the need to work with interpreters and a highly transitory population present unique challenges. Many GPs rise to this challenge and thrive in inner cities. Others, perhaps less well prepared, become despondent and burn out.

■ **Primary care teams**

> Here in the UK there is a primary care system. You are not alone. Back home you are the boss. You tell the patient what to do and what sort of treatment they have to get. What I like here is that you work as part of a team. You work with nurses, social workers, occupational therapists, district nurses, counsellors, dieticians, and you can share the work. In Algeria you do what you can; there is no support.
>
> Otmane El Mezoued, refugee doctor from Algeria

The great majority of GPs work in primary care teams. Team composition and managerial structure vary from practice to practice. Primary care teams provide assessment and treatment of a broad range of conditions, but also have a strong emphasis on promoting health and preventing illness, disease and disability. Primary care teams include all health and social care professionals who deliver community-based care to patients and their families. GP practices, local NHS trusts and social services departments employ different team members. Their work often includes close liaison with charitable and voluntary organisations.

■ Members of the primary care team

GPs
The medically qualified members of the primary care team usually have a strong leadership role. They may be trainers for GP registrars.

GP registrars
These are doctors completing their GP training with a year in practice. They are the equivalent of specialist registrars in hospitals.

Practice nurses
These nurses are based at the practice. They carry out health checks and procedures, including blood pressure measurement, phlebotomy, cervical smears, weight monitoring and contraceptive checks. Many run clinics, for example well woman, smoking cessation, asthma and diabetic clinics.

District nurses
These nurses have undertaken extra training in community nursing. They work in the community, seeing patients in their homes. They change dressings, monitor patients recently discharged from hospital and administer treatment for chronic conditions. They are skilled in a number of specialist assessments, including pressure-sore risk, Barthel scoring, fall risk, incontinence and wound assessments.

Health visitors
Health visitors are nurses with further experience and training in child and family health. They are responsible for improving and maintaining health, and preventing ill health for mothers and children from 10 days after birth (when the midwife hands over care) to four years of age. They provide pre-conception advice on health in pregnancy, and education on breast and bottle feeding, weaning, immunisations and child development, including concerns with walking, talking, sleep patterns and behavioural problems. They also screen mothers for postnatal depression.

Counsellors
Counsellors see people with emotional problems for a time-limited series of regular appointments. Counselling gives patients an opportunity to explore thoughts and feelings in a non-judgemental, supportive relationship. The emphasis is usually on helping people find their own solutions to problems, rather than giving practical help or advice.

Practice manager
The practice manager is the senior administrator in a practice and is responsible for its organisation and administration, as well as supervising reception staff and secretaries. Practice managers have no clinical role.

Reception staff
Reception staff make appointments, organise notes, prepare clinic lists, answer telephones, file letters and investigation results, and are the first point of contact for patients.

Physiotherapists
Physiotherapists manage a range of muscular, bone-related, respiratory and neurological problems and pain.

Dieticians
Dieticians assess and advise patients who require special diets and help them modify their usual consumption. They may, for example, be involved in diabetes clinics.

Social workers
Social workers provide advice, help and support to the elderly, people with learning and/or physical disabilities, people with psychiatric illnesses and children in need of social care services. Services may be provided in patients' homes, day centres, residential centres or, in some cases, foster homes.

Occupational therapists
Occupational therapists help patients who are temporarily or permanently physically disabled as well as others with learning disabilities. They help patients become as independent as possible at home, work and in their social lives. They visit people at home to advise or help with the provision of aids or plan modifications so that a disabled person can get around easily in a wheelchair.

Speech and language therapy
Speech and language therapists specialise in the diagnosis and treatment of speech and language problems, including stammering and vocal or swallowing problems. They see a range of patients from young children with delayed speech to elderly patients who have speech difficulties following a stroke.

Community psychiatric nurses
Community psychiatric nurses (CPNs) specialise in following up and supporting people with psychiatric illnesses. A major part of their work involves helping people with mental illness remain at home, preventing admission or readmission to hospital. They work closely with psychiatrists as well as with GPs. They encourage adherence to care plans and oral medication, administer depot medication and provide a range of therapies.

Community midwives
Community midwives are qualified midwives who may also have undertaken general nurse training. They provide antenatal care in mothers' homes and in GP practices. They visit all newborn babies from discharge from hospital up until the baby is ten days old, and in some circumstances until the baby is six weeks old. They may also undertake home confinements and domino deliveries.

Alternative practitioners
Alternative practitioners such as chiropractors, acupuncture therapists and hypnotists may be part of the primary care team, complementing roles and services provided by traditional practitioners.

■ The new GP contract

GPs have always been self-employed. When the NHS was set up, GPs maintained their independence but registered all their patients and provided 24-hour care for them. This established universal access to GPs for the first time. GPs were paid according to their numbers of patients and also received extra payments for specific activities, including home visits at unsocial hours, maternity care and vaccinations.

GPs working under the new contract (agreed in 2003) may only provide essential care or offer other services, including contraception, vaccination, minor surgery or management of more complex medical conditions.[3] GPs are now able to opt out of providing out-of-hours care.

The new GP contract applies only to GPs working under a general medical services (GMS) contract. It will not affect GPs employed under the personal medical services (PMS) scheme, whose contracts are negotiated locally with primary care trusts (PCTs).

■ PMS and GMS

GPs can work under either locally negotiated PMS contracts arranged with their primary care trusts, or the national GMS contract. PMS contracts aim to improve access to and quality of primary care services, including helping to recruit and retain GPs in areas of greatest need, developing new ways of delivering services, reducing bureaucracy and improving integration of services. Many doctors do not want to wait for parity, invest in premises, take responsibility for employing staff or cover out-of-hours rotas. Women GPs, now more than half the workforce, frequently look for flexible hours to fit in with families. These doctors therefore tend to opt for PMS contracts.

■ References

1 Department of Health (2003) *Statistics for General Medical Practitioners in England, 1992–2002*. The Stationery Office, London.

2 Cross P (2002) The current crisis in GP recruitment. *BMJ*. **325**: S194.

3 Kmietowicz Z (2003) GPs accept contract, but consultants ask for ballot on industrial action. *BMJ*. **326**: 1415.

■ Further reading

Copperfield T (2003) *Tony Copperfield's Primary Care Scream*. Butterworth Heinemann, Oxford.

Cross P (2003) The village GP. *BMJ*. **327**: S101.

Cross P and Rushforth B (2003) A formidable pair. *BMJ*. **327**: S52–53.

Widgery D (1992) *Some Lives: a GP's East End*. Simon and Schuster, London.

CHAPTER 5

Essential paperwork

■ Identification badges

You will need to wear an identification (ID) badge in the hospital or practice. You may need to provide passport photographs for this, or you may be photographed at the hospital, and the image is then printed onto a laminated card. Many cards contain a magnetic strip which provides access to staff-only areas. It may also double as a library card.

■ Contracts

You must ensure that you have a written contract before you start work. This details your duties, pay, annual and study leave entitlements, and start and finish dates. BMA members can send their contracts to the BMA who will check that contracts conform to nationally agreed terms and conditions. This service is included in your membership fee.

■ Annual leave

It is a good idea to arrange and request your leave as far ahead as you can. You will need to complete a leave form, countersigned by your consultant and submitted to medical staffing. When on leave, in most cases colleagues will cover your duties and you will cover for them. It is therefore impossible for everyone to have leave at the same time. Popular times for taking leave are in December (Christmas), April (Easter) and August (school holidays).

■ Study leave

All study leave has to be approved by clinical tutors. Apply well in advance. Doctors use study leave to attend courses and conferences. Some are granted private study leave before postgraduate examinations, but some clinical tutors only grant this if a candidate has been unsuccessful in a previous attempt. Each clinical tutor has a limited education budget for expenses like course fees and travel. Again, a form needs to be filled in when applying for study leave.

■ Clinical paperwork

There was a time when writing in patients' files was a personal matter: a cathartic way of unburdening yourself or an *aide-mémoire* for future reference. It didn't matter if nobody but you could read your scrawl. Not any more. Increasing accountability, patient access to notes and decreased deference to doctors mean what you do and don't write in notes is the difference between being in trouble and vindication.

■ Legibility

How many meticulous clerks are let down by illegible writing? You can't change your handwriting but you can change your pen. Try writing in ink. It is much harder to scrawl using a fountain pen.

■ Identify yourself

A doctor who one of us used to work with had a name stamp. Whenever she wrote in someone's notes, she stamped her name, grade and bleep number in the notes. This might seem excessive or eccentric, but illegible signatures mean many doctors are difficult to identify and contact. GMC guidelines suggest doctors print their name, specialty, grade and bleep number after their signatures. Maybe name stamps will catch on.

■ Pro formas

Clinical note keeping takes time. If you are writing similar information many times for many patients, you might like to consider making a pro forma on a computer. A decision about a patient's resuscitation status can easily be recorded on a pre-printed page of A4 (*see* Box 5.1). These pro formas can be completed during ward rounds. If placed at the front of the notes, nurses will know whether to put out crash calls.

Box 5.1 Example of a pro forma for a patient's resuscitation status

Date:
Name of patient:
In the event of cardiac arrest, this patient is for/not for resuscitation.
Clinical reason:
Patient's wishes:
Discussed with relatives on: [date] [You might like to include a brief summary of discussions with relatives in this section.]
Name of consultant:
Name and grade of doctor completing this form:

Another use of pro formas is in pre-operative administration. A prototype sheet for each common surgical procedure could result in more legible and comprehensive administration. Remember that they are designed to save time and ensure that important questions are asked. However, don't let them turn you into a speaking questionnaire. You can also add extra information to forms. For instance, you might like to record which risks and complications you have warned your patient about.

■ Respect your patients

Patients have access to their medical notes, so it doesn't make sense to write things you wouldn't want them to see. It would be unthinkable to have to explain to parents of a child with dysmorphic features that FLK stands for 'funny-looking kid'.

■ ... and colleagues

It can be tempting to vent clinical and interpersonal frustrations in writing. 'Has still not been reviewed by gynaecologists,' wrote a senior house officer. She wrote it on five consecutive days, underlining 'still' to emphasise her point. The delay turned out to be another miscommunication. The patient had been reviewed on SHO change-over day, but nobody passed the message on. The consultant gynaecologist was angry and wrote a long piece in the patient's notes, in defence of his team. Communications like this hinder good interdisciplinary working.

■ Who was there?

Who was there when you examined Mrs Bloggs? A doctor on a vocational training scheme worked as gynaecology SHO for three months. A year later, a patient he had seen but long since forgotten alleged that he had sexually assaulted her. He had documented that a female medical student was present while he carried out a speculum examination. The medical school was able to trace this particular student, who was able to speak up on his behalf. He said that his only regret was not recording the student's name, as it took several days to work out who it was by a process of elimination.

■ When did this take place?

Always write dates and times in the margins. A family complained to the chief executive that their mother had to wait in casualty for eight hours without seeing a doctor. Her notes stated the times she was seen by three different doctors within three hours of her arrival.

■ Decisions, decisions

Who decided that a 90-year-old demented man was unsuitable for the new 'miracle drug' his grandchildren were demanding? How was that decision reached? Who told his family? Who else was present? How did they react? A few lines suffice:

> *Family meeting: consultant Dr Briggs, SpR Dr Baker, Mrs T Hibberd, grandson Mr Tompkins and granddaughter Mrs French present. Asking for anticholinesterase for pt. Cons. explained not suitable as Lewy-Body dementia. SpR expl. home support available. Introduced to admiral nurse Mrs Hibberd. Visibly upset but understood decision.*

■ Colour

Remember that your notes are legal documents and black ink should usually be used. However, operation notes are traditionally written in red. Green ink is the pharmacists' signature colour. Could colour be used more widely in medical case notes? Abnormal blood results could be circled in red, for example. Bright colours can also be used to highlight management plans, diagnoses and resuscitation status. Unfortunately, colours do not always photocopy well.

■ Handover book

Most doctors hand over details of sick patients to on-call colleagues when they go off duty. Often this information is scribbled on a piece of history paper. There are problems with this. One member of a team might know something specific about a sick patient, but others may not, and the member who does might be on a day off when the sick person deteriorates. Over a bank holiday weekend, up to 20 different doctors may need to know this vital information and the original piece of paper might be lost in a white-coat pocket. Or some information might be remembered and passed from team to team, but gets distorted in the process. This doesn't happen often, but it can take place during busy on-calls. A handover book solves this problem (*see* Box 5.2).

Box 5.2 Example of a handover book

NAME	DoB	WARD	DIAGNOSIS	TO DO
Mrs T	02.05.63	Elmbray	? DVT	Check INR & prescribe warfarin
Mr F	05.08.55	Pineview	COPD	Check ABGs and alter oxygen prescription

---

Handover books need to be kept somewhere accessible. Acute admission or assessment wards are a good place.

Write in nursing notes

Imagine being left nil by mouth for a whole weekend because nurses didn't know you could eat and drink. On a busy ward staffed by many agency nurses, verbal information can be forgotten. One way around this is to write in the nursing notes. Tell the ward manager or sister what you would like to do. As long as your requests are polite and relevant, they usually don't mind and often welcome it.

Joint notes

Joint notes potentially save time and duplication and improve teamwork. Nursing observations are immediately to hand. If relatives have asked to see a doctor and this is in the joint notes, nurses do not need to bleep you. It is often impossible to have a trained nurse on each ward round, especially if there are several consultants sharing a ward, one team on call and one post take and one qualified nurse. Decisions and plans can be read later on.

There are disadvantages to shared notes. Occasionally, nurses will change shift at the same time as a consultant's ward round. A 'tug of notes' ensues: nurses need the notes for handover; doctors need them for the ward round. This game is complicated by true multidisciplinary notes, for example when doctors are unable to write in the notes because a physiotherapist has taken them with the patient to the gym.

Symptomatic relief

Effective clinical note keeping will never be a substitute for clinical competence and all the other qualities that make a complete doctor. But often, clinical records are all that remain when the evidence is buried. The pen might not be mightier than the scalpel, but for those who use one badly, the resultant mess can be almost as lethal.

Discharge summaries

When a patient is discharged from hospital, GPs receive two letters. The first is a pro forma completed by the PRHO or SHO on the day of discharge, usually giving a one-line diagnosis and a list of drugs that have been prescribed. A more complete typed document, the discharge summary, summarising the patient's stay in hospital and aftercare arrangements, is usually written by a more senior doctor and sent to the GP some days or weeks later. Remember, the GP reading the letter may not be the GP who referred the patient. This is particularly true of patients admitted in an emergency or out of working hours. A good discharge summary is helpful to the next doctor to see the patient, as well as to the referring GP, and should contain the following:

- GP's name
- patient's name, address, postcode, date of birth (DOB)
- admission date, discharge date, ward
- consultant's name
- contact name and bleep number for future information
- investigation results
- details of relevant diagnoses, procedures performed, treatments administered
- dates of surgery where relevant
- follow-up care and who will be responsible for carrying this out
- community services already arranged (for example, district nurse, home carer)
- community services that GP needs to arrange
- what patient has been told about the diagnosis
- medication provided on discharge (and how long it is to continue)
- summary of social circumstances.

■ Outpatient letters

Outpatient letters from hospital doctors to GPs are usually written at the end of each clinic session. These are usually dictated on a dictaphone and the tape is passed to the consultant's secretary for typing. Like discharge summaries, outpatient letters are as helpful to your successor in the clinic as they are in keeping the GP updated. They provide snapshots useful for later reviews.

An outpatient letter should include:

- a standard introduction: 'Thank you for referring Mrs Jones' for new patients and 'I reviewed Mrs Smith in clinic today' for patients under review
- summary of demographics: patient's name, address, age and gender. Avoid phrases like 'This delightful 88-year-old lady'
- name and grade of the doctor who saw the patient and the name of the consultant supervising the clinic
- mode of referral
- presenting complaint, history and examination
- investigations carried out and those outstanding
- results of any investigations
- diagnosis or differential diagnosis
- full management details: pharmacological, psychological and social
- natural history of this condition in general and prognosis for this patient in particular
- what the patient has been told
- date of next outpatient review.

■ Using a dictaphone

To be proficient at using a dictaphone takes time. Secretaries appreciate a slow measured delivery. Hold the microphone a hand-width away from your face. Spell out medical terminology and drug names. Start the tape by giving your name, date and a sentence about what the tape contains. You might need to stop and think between sentences; if so, switch the dictaphone onto pause. Find out where spare batteries are kept. Few things are more frustrating than a dictaphone that malfunctions halfway through a busy clinic. Ask secretaries for feedback about your dictaphone technique after you have done a few tapes and act on any recommendation.

■ Copying letters to patients

Sending copies of clinicians' letters to patients is part of the *NHS Plan*.[1] The public inquiry into children's heart surgery at the Bristol Royal Infirmary recommended providing patients with copies of clinical correspondence.[2] This was implemented in April 2004.

Explain to patients that at the end of the consultation you will write a letter to the patient's practice to summarise the main points covered and that they will receive a copy of this letter. Avoid medical jargon unless alternatives are unwieldy or inaccurate. For example, 'Thank you for referring Miss Lynch who has a seven-month history of painful heavy periods' is appropriate for a woman with menorrhagia and dysmenorrhoea. Your trust may have a specific consent procedure and, if this is the case, adhere to it.

■ Writing referral letters

A referral letter must include:

- patient's name and NHS number
- date of birth
- full address, including postcode
- indication of whether the patient needs an interpreter or other special assistance
- name of referring GP.

■ Sick certificates

Patients who are absent from work for less than a week need to complete a self-certificate. These do not require a doctor's signature and are available from the local Department of Social Security (DSS) benefits office. Med 3 certificates are given to patients who have been advised to refrain from work when they are discharged from hospital. You must examine the patient on the day, or the day before, you issue a Med 3. Within the first six months of sickness, a certificate can be issued for up to six months from examination. Certificates issued after the first six months of incapacity can be for any period up to 'indefinite'.

Rules for completing sick certificates
1 Use black ink.
2 Keep blank certificates safe in the same way as you safeguard prescriptions. Blank Med 3 forms could be used fraudulently.

3 Include the patient's name, date of examination and diagnosis which has led you to advise the patient to refrain from work.
4 Don't forget to sign it.

■ Request forms: haematology, microbiology, biochemistry and radiology

Fill in request forms completely. Delays happen when there are discrepancies between information on forms and samples. If you use computer-generated patient labels on request forms, remember to stick one on every page as, unlike your pen, they can't be carbon copied through.

High-risk patients
Don't put your laboratory colleagues at risk. If a patient is at high risk of a blood-borne infection, indicate this in a prominent position on the request form. Similarly, if you are leaving a form for a phlebotomist to take blood from a patient known to have, or to be at high risk of having, a blood-borne infection, you must make sure the phlebotomist knows. Many hospitals have high-risk stickers or an area on the request form that should be ticked.

Urgent blood samples
When making an urgent request, phone the department and discuss the urgency. It may be that the tests can be processed as routine and the results phoned through when available. Sometimes you will need samples processed within minutes and in these cases you must telephone the department and inform staff. Remember to label the request as urgent and add your contact number (bleep or telephone).

■ Prescribing

■ Drug names

Drugs may be known by a trade name, a generic name, or even the chemical group to which the drug belongs. The trade name of a drug varies from one drug company to another, and may also depend on the way in which the substance is formulated for administration or on the country in which it is marketed. In contrast, the generic name, which defines the chemical nature of the substance, does not vary. The trade name may be different from names that are familiar to you from outside the UK. The *British National Formulary* (*BNF*) is useful for checking drug names. You should also be aware that if you prescribe a drug by its generic name, any brand could be dispensed. However, if you prescribe a drug by its trade name, only that brand can be dispensed.

■ The *British National Formulary*

The *BNF* is full of practical and useful advice for safe, effective prescribing. It is published jointly by the BMA and the Royal Pharmaceutical Society of Great

Britain. There are two editions every year (March and September) and it is distributed free to all NHS doctors. You will be able to get a copy from your hospital pharmacist. It is an up-to-date, pocket-sized reference book – independent of the pharmaceutical industry – that gives information on clinical conditions, drugs and other therapeutic preparations. The *BNF* also contains useful information on the practicalities of prescription writing, controlled drugs and dependence, prescribing for children and the elderly, and prescribing in palliative care. Advice is also provided on the reporting of adverse reactions. Prices of each drug are included.

◼ *Drugs and Therapeutics Bulletin*

This is sent free to all GMC-registered doctors every month. It contains helpful updates and advice. If your copy doesn't arrive, phone the medical mailing company on 0800 626 387.

◼ Hospital formulary

Many trusts produce their own formulary, listing drugs available for routine use. They are best used in conjunction with the *BNF*. Hospital formularies are usually regularly updated and monitored by a designated Drug and Therapeutics Committee.

◼ NICE guidelines

The National Institute for Clinical Excellence (NICE) provides guidance on new and existing medicines and treatments, appropriate treatment and care of patients with specific diseases (known as clinical guidelines) and whether intervention procedures used for diagnosis or treatment are safe and efficacious enough for routine use.

Clinical guidelines produced by NICE are colloquially known as NICE guidelines. They are not intended to replace doctors' knowledge and skills. The NICE website contains clinical practice guidelines for a range of conditions and others are continuously being produced: www.nice.org.

◼ Local protocols

Treatment protocols are designed to produce better care at lower cost. Individual trusts often design local protocols because of regional differences in patient populations or available expertise. Their success depends on effective distribution of written summaries of the protocols, ensuring that algorithms are posted in all clinical areas, and reinforcement by pharmacists. It is worth finding out early if there are any local protocols for conditions you will be treating.

■ Hospital prescription charts

The front of a hospital prescription chart will contain spaces for the patient's details and information about allergies. The other sections of the chart include:

- space (usually on the front) for prescribing 'one-off' drugs, for example antibiotics as prophylaxis before an intervention. As well as the dose and administration route, the time and date on which you wish the drug to be given should be entered
- the main part of the chart, for drugs that are to be taken regularly and their doses. This section includes a column for administration times
- a section known as prn, *pro re nata*, which is Latin for as required. Patients or nurses use their own judgement for when these are taken. Specify the dose and a dose interval, such as 'maximum frequency every four hours'. Consider prescribing certain drugs like analgesics and laxatives on the prn side routinely
- a fourth section for infusions. It can be used for fluid management, analgesia and other drugs. The quantity of drug, its reconstitution or dilution, route and rate of infusion should be specified.

Box 5.3 provides a list of common abbreviations used on drug charts.

Box 5.3 Common abbreviations used on hospital prescription charts

Abbreviation	*Meaning*
od	Once daily
bd	Twice daily
tds	Three times a day
qds	Four times a day
prn	As required
stat	To be given immediately
i	One tablet
ii	Two tablets
po	By mouth
pr	By rectum
pv	By vagina
im	Intramuscular
iv	Intravenous
mane	To be taken in the morning
nocte	To be taken at night

Use blue or black ink. Hospital pharmacists use green ink. Hospital pharmacists will do rounds of the ward to inspect drug trolleys and cupboards. They often amend incorrect prescriptions and draw doctors' attention to potential drug interactions. They also mark charts, placing a sticker on each if two patients on the ward have similar names. It is well worth making friends with the ward pharmacist as they will be able to give you advice, up-to-date information and explain the evidence base for different treatments. They will also be able to suggest alternatives for drugs that your patients cannot tolerate.

■ Nurse prescribing

Some nurses are trained to prescribe a limited range of medicines for the following conditions: minor ailments, minor injuries, health promotion and palliative care. Nurses are not allowed to prescribe outside this range of conditions.

■ Verbal orders

In the past, if a doctor could not physically get to a ward, perhaps because they were attending another patient, they would tell a nurse which drug to administer and at which dose and would come to the ward later to sign the prescription chart. Verbal orders can cause problems – nurses may mishear the name or dose, with potentially fatal consequences, and doctors may forget to sign the prescription later – so this method is rarely used.

■ Primary care and community teams

Prescriptions in primary care are written on form FP10. They are taken to high-street chemists to be dispensed.

■ Prescription-only medicines and over-the-counter medicines

Some medicines can be bought over the counter (OTC) at pharmacies, but most are prescription-only (POM), i.e. they can only be dispensed if patients have been given a prescription for them. Patients do not pay for any medication while they are inpatients. Doctors in primary care may advise patients that it is cheaper to buy certain drugs over the counter than to pay prescription charges.

■ Self-prescribing

The GMC recommends that doctors avoid self-prescribing or prescribing for colleagues.

■ Controlled drugs

Drugs that can be misused are called controlled drugs and are subject to the legal requirements of the Misuse of Drugs Act 2001. The *BNF* uses the symbol CD to indicate if a drug is controlled. You must sign, date and write your professional address on all prescriptions for controlled drugs. The following information must also be on the prescription in your own writing:

• patient's name and address
• dosage form (e.g. tablets, syrup)

- total quantity to be dispensed, in words and figures
- dose.

■ Ten tips for safe prescribing

1 Ask patients if they have any drug allergies and what form the allergic reaction takes.
2 Remember that everything that is administered needs to be prescribed. This includes oxygen, fluids, meal replacements and supplements, dressings and bandages, and topical preparations.
3 Involve patients and their carers in discussions regarding changes in medication. Discuss the pros and cons of each treatment, including the expected effects of each treatment as well as adverse effects. Also be honest about the expected effects of no treatment.
4 Neat handwriting minimises errors and confusion.
5 Avoid verbal orders.
6 Don't abbreviate drug names, micrograms and nanograms.
7 Check doses in the *BNF*.
8 Don't leave prescription forms unattended. Lock them away.
9 If you are unsure, ask medical colleagues or the pharmacist.
10 Don't forget to sign prescriptions.

■ Death certification

> I get there and the Blue Bloater's rasped his last breath. I record no pulse under cold clammy skin, no sounds in his chest, nothing but a wide unchanging stare when I shine a light in his eyes. In his notes I pronounce him dead and in the sister's office on the thick pad of death certificates that looks like a giant cheque book, I log the cause of death.
>
> Jed Mercurio, doctor and writer, *Bodies*

In Britain, a death certificate or, more correctly, a 'Certificate for Registration of Death' is the document used to register death. Without one, funerals cannot go ahead. Filling in one of these certificates can be confusing. It is important to do it correctly as errors may result in a delayed funeral and cause further distress to bereaved relatives.

A doctor may only complete a certificate for registration of a death if they have been in attendance to the deceased during the last illness and have seen the deceased within 14 days prior to death or after death. If no doctor meets these criteria, the coroner is informed in England, Wales and Northern Ireland or the procurator fiscal in Scotland.

There are four potential outcomes:

1 an uncertified death
2 death certified by a doctor
3 death certified following a postmortem without an inquest
4 death certified following an inquest.

An uncertified death is very rare, but could occur theoretically. For instance, where a dying patient is attended to before death by a GP who, having discussed the patient with her partners, then emigrates. If such a death is reported to the coroner, they may allow an uncertified death, without requesting a postmortem or inquest. However, in the aftermath of Shipman, this is very unlikely.*

It's worth finding out where death certificates are kept. Usually this is in a bereavement office, but smaller hospitals and general practices have other arrangements. They are contained in a book similar to a large cheque book. There are three sections of paper, separated by perforations. The largest piece is the *Certificate for Registration of Death*, to the left is a *counterfoil* for hospital records that remains attached to the book and on the far right is a *Notice to Informants*, summarising the information.

Ensure you are authorised to complete the death certificate, i.e. you have seen the patient within 14 days prior to death, or after death, and you know the cause. If you are unsure about the cause of death, read through the patient's notes and discuss it with your seniors. If the cause of death remains unclear, it will probably need to be referred to the coroner. Some deaths must be automatically referred to the coroner. These include:

- violent deaths
- deaths when a doctor has not attended in the previous 14 days
- cause of death is unknown or uncertain
- accidental death
- doubtful stillbirth
- deaths related to surgery or anaesthetic
- deaths within 24 hours of admission to hospital.

For some deaths you can issue the Certificate for Registration, but can alert the coroner or other authorities (such as a pension agency) that further action may be required by ticking a box (Box A) on the reverse. Examples of this would be:

- death from an industrial disease
- death of a person who was in receipt of an industrial pension
- death by suicide
- death by poisoning or drugs (including alcohol)
- death as a result of illegal abortion
- death from want, neglect or exposure.

The Certificate for Registration contains the following information:

- Name of deceased
- Age
- Date of death
- Place of death

---

* The late Dr Harold Frederick Shipman was a respected and popular general practitioner in Greater Manchester. He was also a mass murderer who killed up to 250 of his patients by administering fatal injections of morphine. His serial killing, which took place over decades, came to light when police investigated a forged will in 1998.

- Date last seen by the doctor issuing the Certificate for Registration
- This doctor can circle one or more of the following statements:
  - This certificate takes account of information obtained from postmortem
  - Information from postmortem may be available later
  - Postmortem not being held
  - I have reported this death to the Coroner for further action
- There is also an option of one of the following statements:
  - Seen after death by me
  - Seen after death by another medical practitioner, but not by me
  - Not seen after death by a medical practitioner
- Cause of death which is in two parts:
  1a – primary cause of death (and duration, but this is not obligatory)
  1b – due to (and duration, but this is not obligatory)
  1c – due to (and duration, but this is not obligatory)
  2 – significant conditions not related to primary cause of death (can be more than one)
- You can tick Box A if the death is related to employment. It is important to discuss the implications of this with your seniors as it may influence a widow's pension
- Signature of doctor
- Date of issue
- Qualifications of doctor
- The name of the consultant responsible for the deceased if they died in hospital.

Relatives appreciate it if you translate medical terms such as 'myocardial infarction' and 'cerebrovascular accident' into lay terms like 'heart attack' and 'stroke'. It is good practice to put these lay terms in brackets after the medical terms on the *Notice to Informants* section.

■ Example 1

Frieda Smith, a 78-year-old retired school teacher, is registered blind secondary to her diabetic retinopathy and so does not see her dropped novopen on the floor. She falls over it, hurting herself, and is unable to move. Sadly she remains on the floor for three days before being discovered by a neighbour. You are the house officer on call at her local district general hospital. She has fractured her neck of femur and you are instructed to prepare her for theatre. However, she becomes suddenly dyspnoeic and you see that her electrocardiogram (ECG) shows sinus tachycardia. Her arterial blood gases suggest respiratory failure. A VQ scan shows ventilation–perfusion mismatch. Mrs Smith has a cardiorespiratory arrest. You commence CPR and put out a crash call. After 20 minutes' resuscitation, she remains unresponsive and the crash team decide to stop.

Frieda Smith's death certificate:

1a Pulmonary embolus (hours) – you can justify this because of the ECG, blood gas results and VQ scan result. However, uninvestigated shortness of breath three hours before death alone would be no good.

1b Fat embolus (days) – from her fractured neck of femur.
2 Insulin dependent diabetes mellitus (20 years).

■ Example 2

Mrs Mabel Green is 68 years old and is admitted after presenting with pain in her arms, legs and ribs. Her bones are tender and skeletal X-rays show 'punched-out' osteolytic lesions. Bone marrow aspirate contains abundant plasma cells and your team diagnoses myeloma. Mrs Green is treated with chemotherapy but develops renal failure. She and her family ask that she should not be resuscitated in the event of a cardiac arrest. She dies suddenly during one of your nights at work. You suspect she has perished from a hyperkalaemic cardiac arrest.

Mrs Green's death certificate:

1a Tumour lysis syndrome (two weeks).
1b Myeloma (five months).

Remember, you can't give renal failure or cardiac arrest as a cause of death.

■ Example 3

Arthur Pink is a 72-year-old retired docker. Six months ago he was diagnosed with multi-infarct dementia and his wife Grace has been struggling to control his diabetes as he has become reluctant to cooperate with blood glucose monitoring. He has been hypertensive for 20 years, but recently has been forgetting to take his antihypertensives. One morning he falls to the floor and Grace notices that he cannot move his left side. He is admitted to hospital where your team is on call. You diagnose a cerebrovascular accident. Despite treatment and secondary preventive measures, he dies four days later.

Mr Pink's death certificate. In bold in brackets is the sort of lay terminology you might like to include for relatives:

*1a Cerebrovascular accident (**stroke**) (four days)*
*1b Atherosclerosis (**hardening of the arteries**) (five years)*
*1c Hypertension (**high blood pressure**) (20 years)*
2 Diabetes mellitus (ten years)
Multi-infarct dementia (six months)

■ References

1 Department of Health (2000) *The NHS Plan: a plan for investment, a plan for reform*. The Stationery Office, London. www.nhs.uk/nhsplan

2 Public Inquiry into Children's Heart Surgery at the Bristol Royal Infirmary, 1984–95 (2001). In: *Learning from Bristol*. The Stationery Office, London.

■ Further reading

Cross X and Gaunt M (2002) Dictating an outpatient clinic letter. *BMJ*. **324**: S92.

Smith MBH (1998) Can medical students write competent discharge summaries? *Med Teach*. **20** (6): 558–9.

CHAPTER 6

Examinations

■ Revision: don't suffer in silence

Revising alone can be isolating. You are in danger of losing motivation or learning topics less relevant to examinations. Lone learners may struggle for days with concepts that could be explained in minutes by experts.

Revision courses aim to remove tedium from revision. Many promise to teach you all you need to know to pass. They may be informal, run for free by a group of altruistic recent passers. Some informal free courses are advertised but most are known about by word of mouth. Teaching and going through practice questions usually occurs in small groups, where candidates know each other and feel free to ask when they don't understand. However, informality can be a hindrance; for example, the mock exams may feel nothing like the real thing.

Formal revision courses are organised by centres of excellence, district general hospitals with enthusiastic teachers and by commercial organisations or entrepreneurs. Some are organised by Royal Colleges. If you attend a formal revision course, you will usually be provided with handouts, practice questions and other study material. It is also most likely to be able to recreate the anxiety and feeling of a mock clinical or viva voce. It is not uncommon to face these in front of a whole lecture theatre of other candidates. This sounds daunting but if you can survive and learn from it, it sets you in good stead for the exam. Costs vary, but are likely to be in the region of £200 for a weekend course, more if patients are provided for mock clinicals. Revision courses for PLAB and membership exams are advertised in *BMJ Careers*, *Hospital Doctor* and specialties' own journals.

Revision courses aside, don't forget that a normal working week or clinical attachment is packed with potential educational opportunities. Most ward rounds have a teaching component. If you have questions, ask them at the end of the round or between patients, rather than within patients' earshot. Take the opportunity to present cases to SpRs and consultants in exam style and ask for feedback on your performance. Observe cultural differences and language used when doctors gain informed consent or tell patients they have a debilitating disease.

Drug company lunches and meetings give you an opportunity to hone critical appraisal skills. Don't be afraid to ask questions and challenge what is presented. You can learn from representatives (reps) – not by accepting what they say at face value, but by debating with them. It goes without saying that information provided by drug reps invariably favours their products. Draw on your clinical experience and knowledge of research to debunk myths. Playing this game expands confidence in evidence-based prescribing. Warn drug reps when exams are looming. Drug companies often sponsor textbooks and books of multiple-choice questions. You have nothing to lose by being specific and telling reps which part of a particular examination you are sitting.

Junior staff will have protected teaching time. Ask them when this takes place. You may also be able to attend teaching in other departments. For example, if you are doing a surgical clinical attachment and preparing for PLAB part 2, it might make more sense for you to spend one morning attending teaching for A&E SHOs than accompanying the PRHO on ward duties. Be proactive and find out what is going on around the hospital. Asking SHOs from various disciplines directly is a good way to do this. Similarly, if there is an area you are less familiar with, see if you can sit in on an outpatient clinic or attend a ward round. It will set things in context when you read.

Most hospitals have a postgraduate centre where details of educational meetings and talks will be advertised. Ask the centre manager if you can attend those of interest to you. In most cases you will be accommodated. If a consultant you are working with is going to present a paper or address a conference, ask if you can help with administrative jobs. If you arrive early and assist with administration, such as handing out name badges to delegates, it is likely that you will be given a free place.

Online courses and study groups are widely available. Like revision courses they range from those that are free, relying on the goodwill of those running the site, to those run commercially, requiring you to pay to access questions for a fixed time. The free sites may be of poorer quality and are unlikely to be as regularly updated as those run for profit. Commercial courses often have high-quality questions. Look for sites that give answers along with teaching notes or explanations, so that you learn key principles. Online study groups may be good for those too geographically isolated to form a face-to-face group. Like a chatroom, you can visit at your convenience and post questions or advice to others. Beware of rumours, which seem to thrive in online study groups. It is unlikely, for instance, that this is the only place to find out about changes to exam format. If you read something in an online group that you haven't heard anywhere else, it probably isn't true. Go to the GMC or Royal College websites for up-to-date information about exam structure and format.

■ Medical libraries

District general hospitals, teaching hospitals and some larger GP practices and health centres will have a medical library. These vary in size but are particularly useful, especially if there is a medical librarian. Getting them on side is imperative. This is not difficult. Generally, all you need to do is acknowledge every effort they make on your behalf, take the trouble to learn and remember their name, and be particularly grateful when they have gone the extra mile on your behalf.

A library tour may be attached to your hospital induction programme. This is likely to include information on registration, opening hours and borrowing conditions. If, however, there isn't a formal library induction, a polite request should get you a personal tour of the facilities. In today's world this not only includes medical textbooks, journals and periodicals, but also all that is on offer on computers and the internet. Your librarian may be the person to show you how to make a medline search for that obscure paper you need for an audit project. They may also be able to order past papers for exams. It is important to remember that librarians have other responsibilities and will not appreciate having to drop everything just because you need a paper immediately. Librarians often know where you can find things elsewhere even if they haven't got the information to hand. They may be the first point of contact in any research and may search biblio-graphic databases, access electronic publications and online journals on your behalf.

NHS staff may register for an NHS Athens username for access to databases and electronic journals. Even if you are not working in the NHS, you may be able to get an Athens password if you are registered as a student. Athens is a system that allows free access to electronic resources from both work and home. These include full-text electronic journals and clinical databases such as Medline, PsycINFO and Cinahl.

BMA members can use the BMA library. The BMA membership card doubles as a library card. Don't worry if you don't have full GMC registration. EEA doctors applying for registration with the GMC who are members of their national medical association, international doctors who have come to the UK to take a course, or those who have limited registration with the GMC for the period of a training course can all use the library.

For further information contact:

BMA Library
BMA House
Tavistock Square
London WC1H 9JP
Tel: 020 7383 6294
Fax: 020 7388 2544

■ Research and audit

Try to do audit and research as early as you can and get them published. Do talks and presentations. Find ways of making yourself noticed.
Yong Lok Ong, consultant old age psychiatrist from Singapore and Overseas Doctors Dean, London Deanery

When you are designing a project, it is important to understand the differences between clinical audit and research (*see* Box 6.1).

The results of a research project may lead to changes in clinical practice. Audit can be used to ensure changes are implemented. It can also lead to dissemination of important research findings.

Box 6.1: The differences between clinical audit and research

	Research	Audit
Aims	• To generate new knowledge • To test hypotheses	• To identify good clinical practice • To promote health outcomes • To improve service user or carer satisfaction

Methods	• Quantitative research:
	  – randomised controlled trials
	  – cohort studies
	  – case–control studies
	• Qualitative research.
		• Compares clinical practice against evidence-based guidelines or standards
		• Never involves an experimental approach

Data	• Experimental data from clinical trials • Patient notes • Questionnaires • Interviews	• Patient notes • Questionnaires • Interviews
Ethics committee approval	• Almost always required	• Not usually required
Sample	• Usually involves well-defined, often strict selection criteria for participants recruited	• Recruitment criteria not strict
Publication and dissemination	• Usually hopes to publish in a peer-reviewed journal and disseminate results to a wide audience	• Usually local publication, often in the form of a report or presentation

---

■ Higher degrees

Some international doctors wishing to further their education are interested in pursuing a taught postgraduate programme or undertaking research leading to a higher degree of MSc (Master of Science), PhD (Doctor of Philosophy) or MD (Doctor of Medicine).

Most international doctors are primarily interested in clinical training and obtaining a qualification in their specialty, such as membership of the relevant Royal College. In the UK, postgraduate clinical training is organised and examined by the Royal Colleges rather than universities. This is different to many countries where postgraduate training and specialisation is organised and examined by universities.

Experience of research techniques is almost always part of every specialist registrar's experience. However, doctors wishing to pursue an academic career have particular training requirements. Other international doctors may wish to have full-time exposure to and training in research methods, but are not aiming for careers as clinical academics. They are most likely to ultimately work as tertiary care specialists.

Doctors working in lecturer posts usually register for a higher degree and receive specific training in research skills, including data handling, experimental design, statistics, intellectual property rights, health and safety, and research ethics. They usually develop enhanced oral and written communication, IT skills and good time management.

Higher degrees consist of a one-year MSc, an MD with two years of full-time research or a PhD that takes a minimum of three years. While the MD is the traditional research degree for most clinicians, the latter is preferable for those wishing to pursue an academic career.

MSc degrees differ from MDs or PhDs in that they have a structured taught component. MSc courses covering clinical, scientific and more diverse subjects, including teaching, ethics, management and information technology, are widely available. Most MSc courses consist of several modules with a research project and dissertation. Core modules are compulsory but there are usually a number of additional optional modules. An MSc usually involves a year of full-time study, but it is possible to combine it with working as a doctor by attending part time either in the evening or one day a week for two years and preparing assignments in other free time. You will need to have this approved by your employer and tutor before committing yourself.

MD degree structure varies around the UK. Two years of full-time research are required, but this is a minimum and reflects project duration, not time needed for analysis or writing up, for which a maximum of five years may be allowed. It is less formally supervised than a PhD. It may not be recognised in all countries as it is fairly specific to the UK.

A PhD is still the 'gold standard' needed to progress as an academic. It has international recognition. A PhD is always supervised and usually takes three years to complete and longer to write up and submit.

To summarise, international doctors with no aspirations of a career in medical academia, but who do want a higher qualification and enhanced understanding of research methods, would do well to add an MSc to qualifications gained while in the UK. It will also give you an edge over other candidates when applying for SpR training. Clinicians with a strong interest in research may consider applying for an MD, while those committed to an academic career should opt for a PhD.

■ IELTS

The International English Language Testing System (IELTS) tests the English of people who do not speak it as their first language. The examination is jointly managed by University of Cambridge English for Speakers of Other Languages (ESOL) Examinations, the British Council and International Driving Permit (IDP) Education Australia.

All doctors who have qualified outside the UK need to take IELTS before the GMC will grant them registration. The only exceptions are those who are EEA nationals (other than UK nationals) or those with enforceable EC rights.

There are four modules: listening, speaking, reading and writing. Everyone takes the same listening and speaking modules. There is an option to take either academic or general reading and writing modules. However, doctors need to take the academic modules.

■ Marks

Marks are sent out to candidates within two weeks. IELTS provides a Test Report Form giving an ability profile. A score in each module, and an overall score, are recorded as levels of ability called bands:

- There is no pass or fail mark – candidates receive scores on a band scale from 1 to 9.
- In order to sit the PLAB examination you need an overall score of 7 with minimum scores of 7 in the speaking module and 6 in the reading, writing and listening modules. For all other routes to registration you need a minimum score of 7 in all four modules.
- Results are recommended as valid for two years. If your pass in the IELTS test is more than two years old at whichever is the earlier of the date your registration is granted or (where appropriate) the date you passed Part 1 of the PLAB test, you will need to provide proof that you have kept your language skills up to date, or take IELTS again.

■ Explanation of bands[1]

9 Expert user – has fully operational command of the language: appropriate, accurate and fluent with complete understanding.

8 Very good user – has fully operational command of the language with only occasional unsystematic inaccuracies. Misunderstandings may occur in unfamiliar situations. Handles complex detailed argumentation well.

7 Good user – has operational command of the language, though with occasional inaccuracies, inappropriacies and misunderstandings in some situations. Generally handles complex language well and understands detailed reasoning.

6 Competent user – has generally effective command of the language despite some inaccuracies, inappropriacies and misunderstandings. Can use and understand fairly complex language, particularly in familiar situations.

5 Modest user – has partial command of the language, coping with overall meaning in most situations, though is likely to make many mistakes. Should be able to handle basic communication in own field.

4 Limited user – basic competence is limited to familiar situations. Has frequent problems in understanding and expression. Is not able to use complex language.

3 Extremely limited user – conveys and understands only general meaning in very familiar situations. Frequent breakdowns in communication occur.

2 Intermittent user – no real communication is possible except for the most basic information using isolated words or short formulae in familiar situations and to meet immediate needs. Has great difficulty understanding spoken and written English.

1 Non-user – essentially has no ability to use the language beyond possibly a few isolated words.

0 Did not attempt the test – no assessable information provided.

■ Preparing for IELTS

Radio 4 has a lot of programmes about day-to-day problems like congestion charges. You learn English and you learn topical things which helps in your understanding of British culture. Listen to Jeremy Paxman on Newsnight. It gives you a sense of British culture and what's happening in England.

Anonymous refugee paediatrician from Afghanistan

Sit the exam in your home country if you can. IELTS centres are available almost everywhere, from Albania to Zambia. The IELTS website contains a comprehensive list of worldwide test centres and there is probably one near you, although you may have to travel to the country's capital. Having the required IELTS qualification before you get to the UK frees you to concentrate on medicine when you arrive. Phone your local test centre for a list of exam dates. See if you can get hold of an application form at the same time, but don't apply to sit the exam too soon. You need to practise first.

IELTS tests for use and comprehension of the English language. It doesn't test grammar specifically, but you do need to be able to write and speak without making many grammatical errors.

Practise all four components of the exam: listening, speaking, reading and writing.

■ Listening

Listening is the first module to be tested. You will be played a tape and need to write down answers to questions about what you hear. Candidates struggle because it is hard to read questions and listen at the same time. When you practise, get into the habit of writing down answers as you hear them, rather than relying on remembering them until the end of the tape. There will be an opportunity to read the questions through before the tape starts. Do this and underline things on your question paper so you know what to listen out for. Remember you don't need to understand every word of the tape to score highly. There are ten minutes at the end of the listening test to transfer your answers onto a response sheet. You should have all the answers by this stage and can concentrate on presenting them to the best of your ability. Don't leave any gaps on the answer sheet. If you don't know, guess. You might be right.

■ Speaking

The speaking module consists of three parts.

Common topics for part 1 are you, your future plans, reasons for taking IELTS and your home country, family, jobs, hobbies and interests. Practise talking fluently about these subjects and be able to say some interesting things.

In part 2 your examiner will show you a card with a topic on it to discuss. You have a minute to prepare before speaking for about two minutes. They are looking for evidence that you can communicate your thoughts, ideas and opinions, rather than a perfect accent. Try to speak slowly and clearly and look your examiner in the eye. When you are asked to discuss something, think in terms of an essay plan and mention pros and cons of the topic. For extra marks, come to a conclusion, weighing up your arguments. When you have spoken about your topic, the examiner will ask a couple of follow-up questions and move on to part 3.

In part 3 the examiner and you will discuss some more abstract concepts and themes arising from the discussion in part 2. This lasts four to five minutes.

The whole speaking test takes 15 to 20 minutes and will be tape-recorded. If that worries you, practise tape-recording conversations so you are not intimidated on the day. Playing back your recordings can be illuminating and useful as part of your preparation.

■ Reading

In the reading module, you are working against the clock. If you spend too long reading the passage, you won't have enough time to answer the questions. First, read the questions so you know what to look out for when you read the passage. It is well worth spending two or three minutes on this. Second, give yourself a time limit of 20 minutes to read each passage. If you practise reading a passage while looking for answers to specific questions, you will be able to speed read. Again, don't worry about understanding every word or sentence. If you have any time at the end, scan for answers you couldn't find at your first attempt. And guess if you don't know. It won't cost you any marks.

■ Writing

You have an hour to complete two writing tasks. The first typically asks candidates to analyse a chart, graph or table. The second requires you to argue or debate a subject of general and often topical interest. We recommend that you divide the time unequally and spend no more than 20 minutes on the first task and the rest of the hour on the second. You can do them in either order. Try this out when you practise and do what suits you on the day.

You need to write between 150 and 200 words on the graphical information. Many candidates find it difficult to present pictorial information in written form. Introduce the subject. Describe what the chart shows. Is something increasing or decreasing? Are there proportions? Next explain why this might be. If a graph shows that the number of cars going through a major city have decreased but trams have increased, this may be because there has been an increase in car tax, or a toll gate.

When writing the argument or discussion, you will also need to organise information and ideas and write between 250 and 300 words. We suggest you work to a plan such as this:

- Introduction: define all the words in the title and explain what you are going to cover – 50 words
- Arguments for – 100 words
- Arguments against – 100 words
- Conclusion: weigh up your argument; use phrases like 'on balance' – 50 words.

■ Preparation courses

IELTS test centres and language schools offer IELTS preparation courses. We recommend that you attend one. However, quality varies and there may be unscrupulous people after your money. Only attend courses approved by the British Council. They guarantee the quality of courses they endorse. Their website www.british council.org has details of courses worldwide.

IELTS website www.ielts.org contains a lot of useful information and sample material. You can also download the IELTS handbook in pdf format for free.

■ PLAB

■ The low-down

PLAB, the Professional and Linguistic Assessments Board examination, is conducted by the GMC and supported by the British Council which organise and administrate PLAB part 1 exams outside the UK. It is designed to assess overseas doctors' ability to work safely as an SHO in a UK hospital and is a prerequisite for most overseas doctors' GMC registration. Every year, about 12 000 doctors sit PLAB.

■ Part 1

Part 1 is a written paper, usually taken in the candidate's home country. Examiners expect doctors to have the breadth of knowledge needed to qualify from medical school supplemented by a year's experience as a pre-registration house officer. Currently the paper consists of 200 extended matching questions (EMQs).

■ Part 2

Part 2 is an objective structured clinical examination (OSCE). This tests clinical and communication skills in 14 stations. At each station you carry out a task. This may be talking to or examining a patient, demonstrating a procedure on an anatomical model for example suturing, phlebotomy or resuscitating a dummy. You are awarded an overall A, B, C, D or E at each station. As long as you don't get a D at more than four stations or an E at two, you will pass. There are 16 stations in total, but there is a rest station and a pilot station where new questions are tested. Marks from the pilot station do not count towards the exam. You must pass part 2 within two years of passing part 1.

■ How much does it cost?

Part 1: £145
Part 2: £430

■ Who writes the questions?

The GMC advertises for a panel of writers. Interested doctors are invited to a question-writing day where they are taught how to write effective questions. These are written by a GP with a surgeon, a psychiatrist with a paediatrician and a physician with an obstetrician to prevent them writing effete questions at specialist level. Questions are written in the morning and in the afternoon the groups swap and check the style and format of the other group's questions. If they don't understand the question, or think it too difficult, it gets scrapped.

■ Pass rate

The part 1 pass rate varies, but is usually somewhere in excess of 60%. The pass rate for part 2 is around 70%.

■ Examiner's advice for part 1

Professor Kenneth Cochran advises candidates to work from general textbooks used by UK medical schools (*see* Further reading at the end of this chapter): 'There are no hidden traps. People who become specialised find the exam hard because it is at the very general level of a recent medical graduate.

We ran a pilot on UK graduates coming to the end of their PRHO year. We asked them about timing and appropriateness of questions. Those are the questions we are using now. It's not obscure knowledge. It's more like "a mother brings a child who has a rash".'

■ Examiner's advice for part 2

Dr Malcolm Campbell, chairman of the part 2 panel, says: 'We are looking for basic clinical competence at the level of a first-day SHO in any specialty. Candidates shoot themselves in the foot by rote learning and by going to these dreadful crammers. Many learn the right questions and don't listen to patients' answers. For example, the doctor says to a simulated patient "How are you feeling?" and the simulated patient says "I think I'm going to kill myself", and the doctor says "And how are your bowels?".

I would recommend people try to scrape together enough cash to spend a month in the UK doing a clinical attachment. This would serve two purposes: they would pick up a lot of how medicine is done in the UK and it improves medical language skills, making them confident.

Our simulated patients are trained to behave like real ones. A lot of candidates are taken aback when patients ask questions like "Why should I do this?", "What are the side effects of this?" and "Is that the best course of action?". We are not suggesting that the way we interact is better, but that is the way that patients are dealt with in the UK.

We don't expect candidates to be brilliant, rather the kind of doctor a consultant can trust to know their limitations, make basic diagnoses and not kill too many patients. We are not looking for perfection. Everybody makes mistakes.'

■ Advice from candidates

Mohammad Amjad Khan sat PLAB part 1 in Pakistan: 'I used several different study methods: studying on my own, in a group and using past papers from the market. The hardest part was subspecialty EMQs on skin diseases, orthopaedics and psychiatry. With the benefit of hindsight, I would not have relied on Indian EMQ books from the market as most of them were substandard and not clinically relevant.

Stick to EMQ books written by UK authors such as Una Coles.[2] If you can find a partner to study with, it is worth anything. I recommend the Medic Byte PLAB 1 Course (www.medicbyte.com) as well as the PasTest EMQs.[3]'

Archana Mischra from north India is a paediatric SHO in Manchester. She passed PLAB part 2 and remembers: 'Once you know the system you just fly through. But if you don't know how to approach it, or what you are expected to do, you're sure to fail.'

A refugee surgeon from the Congo who preferred to remain anonymous feels: 'In my country I spent a long time training in surgery and to pass PLAB you have to be good at everything, even things you read ten years ago at medical school. Go back and learn them again. I go to a study group for refugee doctors at Queen Mary College which teaches you how things are done in the UK, and that's what we need for part 2.'

Otmane El Mezoued, a refugee doctor from Algeria, explains some of his difficulties with PLAB: 'In Algeria we had to write essays. In this country there are MCQs, EMQs and OSCES. You have to learn exam technique. I didn't pass PLAB 1 the first time. I thought books would be enough but even if you are a genius and try to do PLAB without practising EMQs, you will fail. Go to any PLAB centre and wait for people who have just done the exam. Ask them when they come out where the study groups are. I joined a study group and passed.'

Otmane also encountered some cultural difficulties with the OSCE: 'For part 2 there may be a station on how to break bad news. If you don't know the culture and how people react to bereavement, you will fail. In the UK, you involve patients in management decisions and they have the right to know what is wrong with them. In Algeria, if a patient has cancer, you talk to the family and they decide whether to tell the patient. The family makes those decisions, not the clinician. Be careful with body language. If you come from a Mediterranean country you use more hand gestures, which UK patients might interpret as aggressive. I have problems controlling my hands. Now I clasp my hands together and interlink my fingers. Make yourself familiar with how UK hospitals run. What are the protocols? How do you take blood? How do you put a urinary catheter in? If you don't see how people do it in this country, you are in trouble.'

A refugee paediatrician from Afghanistan who also wished to remain anonymous describes his frustrations with PLAB: 'I did a driving test here and passed on my fourth attempt. PLAB is like a driving test. It is about doing things in a certain way. I took PLAB so many times I gave up and just left it. I realised I was knocking at a closed door, but I had to keep on knocking. If you want to make it, keep knocking. I went back and sat it and passed.'

■ Essentials for PLAB part 2

Clinical skills

Make sure you are competent at the following clinical skills: examining respiratory, cardiovascular, abdominal and neurological systems; examining joints; vaginal examination, including taking a cervical smear; fundoscopy; taking blood; inserting an intravenous cannula; inserting a urinary catheter; inserting a nasogastic tube and checking its position on an X-ray; and blood pressure measurement.

Communication skills

Practise obtaining informed consent to common procedures. Be able to explain clinical conditions in layman's terms. You should be able to break bad news for a variety of conditions, including motor neurone disease, multiple sclerosis and cancer.

Ten tips for the OSCE

1 Introduce yourself and be courteous to patients.
2 Read or listen to instructions carefully.
3 Ask for permission before examining and explain the procedure, even if you are examining a dummy.
4 Offer patients choice. If you are asked to take blood, ask which arm they would prefer you to use. If you are required to give them information, establish what they know and ask if they have any questions.
5 Don't hurt your patient. For example, if the patient has abdominal pain, start palpating in an area that is not painful. If pain is unavoidable, for instance when you are taking blood, warn the patient beforehand. Say something like 'Sharp pain coming now'.
6 Look first. There may be clues around like a hearing aid, asthma inhaler or colour chart telling you what blood bottles to use.
7 Describe physical findings before giving a diagnosis.
8 Look the examiner in the eye. Speak confidently. Don't mumble or look at the floor.
9 Don't dwell on a bad station.
10 Thank patients and examiners at the end of each station.

■ How to pass membership exams

Membership exams are hard. Royal College pass rates vary, but are around 50%, so you need more than talent and luck. You need a strategy.

■ 1 Decide when to sit the exam

Prioritise. Juggling half-hearted revision with busy working days, home or office paperwork and flat hunting is bad news. Unlike undergraduate exams, you can choose when to sit memberships exams. Of course you can't put them off forever, but the right time for colleagues may not be for you.

■ 2 Pick a start date

Once you have selected a time, apply to sit the exam. Closing dates can be very early and you need to send your application form and passport photos to the examinations department of the Royal College. Decide on the date you will start revision and circle it on the calendar.

■ 3 Warn family and friends

You are going to become an exam bore. Warn your loved ones that you are about to become obsessed with medical minutiae. You will panic, fret and snap at those who least deserve it. Spare-time revision requires discipline. You will need to ignore the clamours of children, nagging flatmates and household chores. If no one else mends it, the tap will have to drip.

■ 4 Recruit colleagues

Revision shared is revision halved. Working in a group has advantages. A bigger pool of MCQs, OSCE stations and a greater collection of patients with interesting signs are important examples, but perhaps more importantly, you get a chance to benefit from other doctors' training and experience. An ideal study group size is four or five people – any less and you can be tempted to put off revision. Larger groups tend to waste more time. Avoid the temptation to revise exclusively with other overseas doctors. Studying with British-trained graduates will give you an insight into the expected balance between book knowledge and practical skills. If no one else in your hospital is sitting the exam, consider joining an online study group.

■ 5 Before your start date

Like an athlete, you need decent kit. Essentials include pads of punched A4 paper, pens and highlighters. You need little books crammed with key facts. There are many in print and rather than fight over a few library copies, buy a few. But don't buy more than one for each topic. Spend a Saturday afternoon getting your stationery and books so you don't waste revision time later panic-buying fat reference books that you will never have time to read.

■ 6 Months before the exam

Know your enemy. Get hold of as many past papers as you can. This gives you insight into your examiners' minds. While exams are meant to test breadth of knowledge, there are some topics which lend themselves to testing in MCQ, best-of-five (BoF) and individual statement questions (ISQ) formats, others to essay format. If your College produces a syllabus, write to them and request a copy. If not, past questions are a useful indication of likely topics. Speak to people who have just passed and borrow their revision materials from them. Some exams require you to produce a logbook, case commentaries or dissertation. Resist the temptation to leave these to a last-minute search of written-up and mislaid cases.

Writtten exams are usually set six months before you sit them. Look at the *BMJ*, *Lancet* and a couple of your specialty's major journals published six months ago. This gives you an idea of what was topical. If any important advances have been made, evidence-based guidelines published or legal history changed, make brief notes of these with a date, journal and author names. With practice, you will be able to drop these references into essays, short-answer questions, long-case discussion and viva voces.

Clinical examinations provoke anxiety. If you have an accent, it may be difficult for examiners to understand what you are saying. This is particularly true if you speak quickly when under pressure. Ask friends to be examiners and practise answering mock questions.

■ 7 Weeks before the exam

If you use public transport, take self-test and revision fact books with you. If you drive, read revision notes into a tape recorder and listen to it on the way to work. Start revising at work: a few MCQs for every patient who DNAs in clinic; practise your viva technique with the SpR for ten minutes at the end of every ward round. As you revise, you will come across topics of which you are ignorant. Keep a list of these. It can be comforting to go over familiar and easy material, but you must get this list out and ask your study group and seniors to help you.

Take all the study leave you can. Study leave is discretionary, but the BMA recommend periods which trusts usually incorporate into contracts. Typically, SHOs are recommended to have up to 30 days per year and SpRs either day-release equivalent of one working day per week during university terms or up to 30 days per year. Exam days should not be taken out of this entitlement.

Your logbook, case discussions or dissertation should be typed and bound. If you are behind, consider paying to have it done professionally. Go on a revision course. They get through a lot more material than if you revise alone. You will feel motivated and come back with handouts to consolidate new knowledge. They are expensive, but so are resits. Approach speakers with specific questions over lunch. Speak to someone who has failed. Find out where they went wrong and learn from their mistakes.

A key to examination success is being able to organise your answer. For example, a plan for any essay question is:

- define all terms in the title
- describe the essay's aims
- present arguments in favour
- present arguments against
- weigh up arguments and conclude by either quoting someone else, criticising the title or looking to the future.

■ 8 Days before the exam

Reread your course handouts and quotations. Redo some tricky questions and make sure you understand them. There will still be a few things that don't stick. Aim to get them onto a page of A4. Read it every night. Make sure you know how to get to the examination venue.

■ 9 Exam day

Generally people fall into two categories: last-minute crammers sitting outside exam halls, hours early, reading pages of notes and last-minute arrivals who run in as the papers are being given out. There is a third way. Get there in good time but no more than an hour early. It's too late to learn anything new. Buy a newspaper. It gives a sense of perspective and will tune your brain into English if this is not your first language.

■ 10 Viva voce survival

'The examiners just want to have a sensible conversation with a colleague about the case.' Have you heard this about vivas? It's rubbish. This is not the time for exchanging pleasantries. You are being examined for a competitive exam. There is a fine line between showing off, leaving the examiners feeling patronised by an arrogant candidate, and on the other hand appearing too uncertain to make clinical decisions. Speak sensibly but with authority, for example: 'I would do X as described by Hodges.'

■ 11 Limbo

All exams involve a period of limbo while you wait for results or have a gap between written and clinical exams. Either way, you deserve a few days off. If you have a few weeks before clinicals, you will have enough theoretical knowledge from the written papers but need to see loads of patients. Remind senior staff that you need exam practice. Somewhere within commutable distance there may be a friend of a friend who is a college examiner. Track them down and ask for exam practice. Ask them why candidates fail and if there are any particular pitfalls for overseas doctors.

■ 12 And if at first you don't succeed

Remind yourself that this is an unfair, subjective system and look at all the good doctors you know who had a second or even third bite at the Royal College cherry. Your family and friends will be glad to have more of your time. Forget about exams for a while so when you do reapply you start your revision refreshed.

■ MRCP
■ The low-down

The MRCP (Member of the Royal College of Physicians, London) part 1 examination consists of two 'best of five' (candidates choose the best answer from five answers) papers, each lasting three hours. These questions test a wide range of common or important disorders. In part 2, two written papers contain up to 100 'best of five' questions. All questions include a clinical scenario.

If you pass both written sections, you can sit the Practical Assessment of Clinical Examination Skills (PACES). The PACES examination consists of five clinical stations, each assessed by two independent examiners. Candidates start at any station, before moving onto others at 20-minute intervals. Part 2 must be completed within seven years of Part 1.

■ How much does it cost?

Part 1 examination: £285
Part 2 written examination: £285
Part 2 clinical examination (PACES): £450

There is an additional £180 diploma fee before you can put MRCP after your name.

■ Who writes the questions?

The Royal College of Physicians' Specialty Question Groups devise new questions.

■ A candidate's story

Mark Westwood is a cardiology SpR at Barts and The London. He passed part 1 first time, but passed part 2 on his second attempt. He frequently helps SHOs preparing for MRCP, sharing his successful formula.

Part 1
'The part 1 syllabus looks like the first year of medical school, only 20 times harder. Three months before part 1, I bought lots of MCQ books and ploughed through them. I went on the Pastest course four months before the exam. I recommend going on a revision course early as it showed me how much work there was. On the Pastest course I was given a folder of questions which previous candidates have memorised, so when I sat the exam I had seen some of the questions before. Examiners may change the question slightly, but if someone has explained it to you and you understand what you are being asked, you are likely to score very well. Candidates' mark distributions are so close that probably all you need to pass is some past questions. Read and learn *The Complete MRCP Part 1: MCQs* by Hugh Beynon.[4] He's a clever bloke. His questions are very difficult but the explanations are superb, and you will learn a lot about weird and strange diseases

that creep up because examiners like asking about them. It gives you an insight into how questions are written.'

Part 2

'I recommend Sanjay Sharma's *Rapid Review of Clinical Medicine* for part 2.[5] It got me through the written, but I messed up the clinical. If a station goes badly it can mar the whole exam. The clinical component is unbelievably stressful and it is easy to muddle up clinical signs. If examiners are watching you and ticking boxes it is very easy to do badly because it isn't the same as real life. I don't think any clinical exam is like real life.'

Pass rates

'They only let a third of people pass at each sitting. The vast majority of candidates are doing busy district general hospital jobs and cram their revision around that. Most people will pass, just not at their first sitting.'

PACES

'Keep your head during PACES. As you do each station, forget the previous one. Even if you have said something silly, like mentioning a collapsing pulse on a patient with aortic stenosis, forget it. When I failed it was because I was thinking about something I did wrong for the next half-hour. Move on and do your best, over and over. I did that the second time. It worked.

Stress

'Each time you sit the exam it exposes you to extreme stress, which gets easier to deal with. Courses recreate mock PACES, but because you know it's a mock, however mean and horrible your examiners act, it is nothing like the big day.'

Final advice

'This is going to be one of the most miserable periods of your life. You are working very hard and being a student in your spare time. It feels like a treadmill and that's exactly what it is. Remember you may not pass this time, but if you are determined you will get the MRCP in the end.'

Claire Collett also took more than one attempt before passing the MRCP at the end of last year. She recommends 'doing a bit each day and finding someone to revise with as you can motivate each other. I did thousands of MCQs for part 1. For part 2 I did lots of book work, but with hindsight feel that Ryder's *An Aid to the MRCP Short Cases*[6] and Baglia's *250 Cases in Clinical Medicine*[7] are the only books worth getting. I revised for PACES using these two books and by seeing lots of patients. The first time round I got too nervous to think for the PACES exam.'

■ An examiner's experience

Dr Neil Dewhurst is an experienced examiner for the MRCP: 'Most UK candidates will be on an SHO rotation and after 18 months should be able to get through the MRCP. Some do part 1 after house jobs, but the fastest to the final clinical is two and a half years. We are looking at a doctor of that vintage.'

Part 1

'Part 1 has a pass rate of 35%. It's tough. Many doctors underestimate the scope of clinical knowledge expected. They are unprepared. We may not want incredible detail, but we do want breadth.'

Written exams

'Best of five questions test basic science as well as statistics, clinical pharmacology and other specialties – areas that give specialist registrars the knowledge base and powers of deduction to use basic information in clinical settings.

Part 2 has a pass rate of 60–65%. Candidates tend to trip up on interpretation of scientific information.'

Obstruction

'The College isn't being obstructive by producing an exam which is too difficult or irrelevant. Any assessment will be flawed, but there has to be some sort of written assessment and it has to be wide-ranging.'

Revision courses

'Preparation takes months. Crammer approaches are difficult to uphold educationally. There are always instances in PACES where you see they've been taught this way or that way.'

Textbooks

'We use the *Oxford Textbook of Medicine* as our reference.[8] If it isn't in there then it won't be in the exam. We don't look for obscurity.'

Professor Peter Kopelman is the incoming chairman of the MRCP Clinical Examining Board. His area of expertise is PACES.

PACES

'Station 1 is on the respiratory system and abdomen. There is an introductory spiel like: "This 44-year-old man gives a three-month history of progressively worsening shortness of breath." Just as in real life there might be patients without physical signs. At six minutes candidates are warned that there is one minute left, after which they are asked to present findings and discuss management and investigations. After ten minutes, candidates move to a patient with abdominal problems.

The candidate has five minutes outside station 2 for history taking. They read a GP letter, for example: "Dear Dr, I'm very concerned about this patient who has had an increase in bowel motion and is passing blood." They then carry out a task in the letter, like "give your opinion". At 14 minutes the patient leaves: the candidate has a minute to reflect and examiners ask questions.

The candidate then goes to station 3 and faces a ten-minute examination of a patient with a cardiovascular problem and ten minutes with a patient with a neurological problem.

Station 4 is the communication station. It may be breaking bad news, explaining a procedure to a patient or relative, or explaining withdrawal of feeding or a decision not to resuscitate. My colleagues and I vet scenarios before they are used. We rehearse scenarios with simulated patients and agree what a doctor should do. We are trying to replicate real life.

The last station includes other systems: eyes, skin and locomotion. Candidates are asked what they find and how they would investigate and manage, so it is more than just a spot diagnosis.

Candidates fail because they have poor examination technique or poor history-taking skills. Others are unable to interpret findings to put together a differential diagnosis. Increasingly, young doctors are aware that revision courses only tell you about exam method, and that application and interpretation of physical signs come from experience.

My advice to candidates is to be as experienced as you can. Go back to day one of medical training and read a clinical methods book. Appreciate the applied physiology. Understand what physical signs mean. A lot of junior doctors are poor at analysing them. Be observed in your clinical method by a senior doctor who is prepared to compliment or criticise. Courses can't provide that but the consultant on your post take ward round can.'

■ MRCS

■ The low-down

There are three components of the intercollegiate MRCS (Member of the Royal College of Surgeons, England) examination:

* part 1: applied basic sciences MCQ paper
* part 2: clinical problem solving MCQ paper
* part 3: viva voce and clinical examinations.

Despite the apparent distinction, the applied basic sciences paper includes clinical knowledge, especially in application of basic sciences, and some clinical problem-solving questions require knowledge of basic sciences. Under new regulations, the entry requirements to parts 1 and 2 are that candidates must have a primary medical qualification acceptable for full or limited GMC registration and have started basic surgical training. This means you can sit the MRCS at any point during basic surgical training. Candidates have three and a half years from their first attempt at part 2 to complete all parts.

■ How much does it cost?

Parts 1 and 2: £175 each
Part 3 Oral costs: £320
Part 3 Clinical costs: £330

Candidates passing all sections have to pay an admissions fee of £100 before they can use the letters MRCS.

■ Who writes the questions?

Questions are drawn from college question banks.

■ Pass rate

'Our pass rates are quite high,' says Ruth Palmer, head of the examination department. 'For MCQ papers typical pass rates would be 70%, for the vivas 40% and the clinical 60%. Communication skills pass rates are between 70–80%.'

■ The examiner's view

'We're not trying to assess whether candidates have a particular attitude,' explains Ruth Palmer, 'but there are competencies we are looking for. For the clinical we want them to conduct a systemic clinical examination. To know that they can discuss investigations, diagnosis and management. In the vivas we are looking for candidates to be able to apply their knowledge and present it in a well-organised manner.'

Ruth runs through reasons candidates commonly fail: 'Insufficient preparation for MCQs and an inadequate knowledge base for the vivas. Many candidates haven't revised enough. There are gaps in their knowledge or they can't apply what they have learned. People fail the clinical because they take it too soon. They haven't had enough experience. The other reason for failure is insufficient structured training.'

Denis Wilkins, Chairman of Examiners, explains that doctors run into difficulty when they have not been in good training posts: 'Try by word of mouth to find good jobs where you will actually be given some training as opposed to being a pair of hands with very little training,' he advises. 'This may involve speaking to people doing the post as well as the human resources (HR) department.' He feels this can be a particular problem for overseas doctors and suggests they 'obtain support and sponsorship from someone who has connections with this country. Many doctors from abroad have a good grasp of factual knowledge, in many cases better than British trainees.'

■ The candidate's view

Ben Challacombe, clinical research fellow in urology at Guy's Hospital, London, explains the changes to the MRCS: 'They've changed format to link all Royal Colleges together. The MRCS is taken after basic surgical training. There are time limits when you can take the jobs, which previously were 20 and 22 months for the clinical and the viva, respectively. And the way they used to have it was that you did the viva first and the clinical second. They reversed that last year. Prior to that there are two multiple-choice papers which contain multiple-choice and extended matching questions. They used to be run by the four different Colleges; the current plan is to bring all the Royal Colleges together and for you to do one generic exam. In the past your degree would say MRCS (England), MRCS (Glasgow), MRCS (Dublin) or MRCS (Edinburgh).'

Ben prepared for the MCQ papers by working as an anatomy demonstrator: 'I would advise doing it. It means anatomy and physiology suddenly become second nature. Instead of cramming it all in, actually teaching anatomy means you learn it.' He also did a 'vast number of MCQs. You need to do four or five thousand questions.'

For the clinical and viva examinations, Ben did an MRCS clinical and viva course at St Thomas' that was run by Pastest. 'There are also very good ones at Whipps Cross,' he adds. 'The Whipps Cross course has been going for 30 years. It's a three-week course and it's absolutely brilliant. You watch the consultant examining people, as they would like you to do in the exam. You're lectured on the various elements of the viva, which is in three basic science areas and three clinical areas: anatomy, physiology, pathology, intensive care, principles and practice of surgery, and operative surgery. Those are the six areas you're vivaed on.'

Ben also found it useful to sit in on outpatient clinics: 'I did a general surgery clinic, orthopaedics clinic and spoke to an ear, nose and throat (ENT) person about how to examine that system. It's important to get your boss to watch you examine someone to ensure you're doing it right.'

'Make it like the driving test,' he suggests. 'Start with a set sequence of things to get maximum points. My mnemonic is IPEEP, which stands for Introduction, Positioning of the patient, Explanation of what you are going to do, Exposure of the patient and Privacy of the patient and asking if they have any pain. These exams are marked on a mark sheet. Although you can get the answer to what the diagnosis is, you can still fail the examination for not getting ticks in all the right boxes. You have to nail it by saying: "Hello sir, my name's Ben Challacombe. I'm one of the doctors here. Can I have a look at you? Would you mind lying flat for me?" Telling the examiner, "Ideally I'd like to expose this gentleman from the knees to the armpits for this examination. I'm just going to shut the door for privacy, and ask if there is any tenderness or pain, and let him know that if I do cause him any discomfort of course I'll stop." That line is useable for any examination. Also look round the bed in an exaggerated fashion for points and clues like a walking stick, oxygen mask, glasses, sputum pot or inhaler. If there are 45 treatment cards it suggests that the patient has been in hospital a while. When you've done IPEEP, stand back at the end of the bed in a way you'd never do in practice and move your head up and down and back and forth as though you're looking around the bed. Then look at the patient as a whole – because there is a mark for that – and then start the actual examination. Likewise, at the end say "Thank you very much, sir", making sure that they are sitting back up, and help them put their clothes back on. There's another couple of marks there. If you just come in and feel the lump in the tummy, you're unlikely to pass.'

Ben believes the viva voce is the most nerve-wracking component of the exam: 'The best thing is to practise with colleagues. It can be quite lonely. It's not like revising for finals when you've got the whole year. It's important to find another chap or chapess to do the exam with. You can revise a bit, go over it again, meet up and ask each other questions. Viva each other in a nasty way so it's better when you get to the real thing. Revising on your own is much more difficult.'

The book that helped Ben prepare for the viva is *General Pathology Vivas* by Lowe.[9] 'That was the best book,' he says, 'because it has nightmare vivas you'd never think of. Ones that if you got in an exam you'd completely fall apart. Look at each page of this book and you will always be able to say something to bail yourself out of trouble. There are quite bizarre things you'd never see in clinical practice that they love asking about.'

■ MRCGP

■ The low-down

The MRCGP (Member of the Royal College of General Practitioners) is a credit accumulation examination. Candidates must pass four modules within three years, or retake the whole exam.

The four modules are:

- a written paper
- a multiple-choice paper
- an assessment of consulting skills by one of two methods:
  - video recordings of consultations
  - 'simulated surgery', in which a series of standardised patients are portrayed by role-players. This is only available to those candidates who have insuperable difficulties making videos. In practice this means people who have finished their training and are working as locums. Pitching up and asking 'Do you mind my video?' may not be a practical option. Others may have religious objections to videotaping patients
- an oral examination.

You don't have to pass one module before sitting the next, and each is available in summer or winter.

■ Components and requirements

You can sit the examination if you are eligible to be an independent GP, or if you are undergoing vocational training. This means a GP registrar embarking on their vocational training is entitled to sit the MRCGP from the day they start. Most do it towards the end of training.

You must provide evidence of proficiency in cardiopulmonary resuscitation.

■ How much does it cost?

£275 per module

■ Who writes the questions?

A panel of practising GPs, recruited by the College, write all questions.

■ Pass rate

The pass rate is 80%.

■ Multiple choice

The three-hour MCQ paper has 200 items: 65% is on medicine, 15% on administration and management, and 20% on research, epidemiology and statistics. Traditional true/false questions have been replaced with single best answers where you have a choice of five responses arising from clinical vignettes. Extended matching questions, where clinical scenarios are followed by a number of options, are also included.

■ Construct marking

For the written paper, examiners predetermine so-called constructs that they look for in candidates' answers. Candidates don't know what the constructs are. However, the college website contains specimen answers, giving a good idea of the constructs they are looking for.

■ Video

The video is a test of consulting skills. Examiners are looking for doctors who encourage patient contribution, respond to cues and elicit details, placing a complaint in a social or psychological context.

■ Oral exam

This comprises two 20-minute orals conducted by two examiners with a break of five minutes. The oral examination is structured to look at professional values underpinning decision making. Examiners are searching for evidence that the candidate's decision making is rational, ethical and sensitive. There isn't always a correct answer. Certain areas like patient care, working with colleagues, the social role of general practice and the doctor's personal responsibility are favourites.

■ The examiner's view

David Sales is Deputy Conveyer of the MRCGP: 'All 150 examiners are practising GPs. We do not trick candidates. Every question is something a jobbing GP will come across. The simple reason people fail is that they are not good enough. In the written paper candidates are presented with clinical material or material relating to a drug trial and asked to integrate, evaluate and synthesise answers. For example, a question in a recent paper was "The Boulderson family of five has had 12 out-of-hours visits during the past month. What issues does this raise?" We are also looking for the ability to use critical appraisal skills and to reapply that in practice. In another recent paper we presented data comparing Effexor® and fluoxetine. Candidates were asked how drug company literature differs from a scientific paper.

The video upsets candidates the most. There is a tendency for candidates to put a list of the performance criteria up in front of them when they are consulting and to just go through the tick-list in a non-thinking manner. They do it in a way that is almost rote performance. Each tape is marked by seven examiners, independent of each other, judging performances against predetermined criteria. We want active listening and open-ended questions. Candidates should demonstrate that at the end of a consultation they know more about that patient than at the beginning. We also hope candidates will be able to explain a diagnosis in words of one syllable.

In the oral we ask questions such as "What makes an effective primary care team?", "How would you communicate with the media?", "How would you deal with aggressive patients?", "What do you do if patients bring you a gift?", "How does it make you feel?" and "Do you accept it?". If candidates have a superficial appreciation of ethical issues, or they can't discuss topics in depth, then we start getting worried.

People who revise with study buddies or work in groups do better. Critical appraisal skills, hot topics and new question formats are readily available on courses, including those that the College runs, but a lot of other commercial organisations, deaneries and facilities offer courses throughout the UK. They are variable but they offer practice exams – and the more of those that you can do, the better.'

The future

'We're looking at an assessment package which integrates workplace-based performance. There will be a test of competence which is going to be a knowledge test, which may be machine markable. There may be an OCSE using either real patients or simulated ones. It's not firmed up yet but exams are evolving.'

■ The candidate's view

Attiya Khan has just passed the MRCGP and completed her GP registrar year: 'People say GP exams are easy. Compared to other postgraduate exams they have a much higher pass rate. I failed the MCQ first time. I didn't do enough book work and underestimated how hard it was.'

Exam technique

'The RCGP website has practice written papers and sample answers that are useful. Go on a RCGP course. They are really expensive, but if you don't you'll find it difficult to pass. They give you questions like: "Daisy Boyd, aged 69, presents to your surgery smelling of urine. What do you do?" Most people say they will do a history examination and investigations, and for that they get five marks out of a possible 25. The RCGP want you to say: "According to this consultation framework, these are the issues for the patient, issues for the doctor, issues for the practice and issues for society." Ask yourself, "Why has the patient come at this point? What is going on in her life?" Give a plan of the history, examination and investigations and what impact this has on your practice. Mention time constraints and what referral facilities you have. For Daisy Boyd, you need to discuss the ageing population and her inadequate care as well as cost implications.'

Hot topics

'In the written paper there is a section called hot topics and you need to know the last 18 months of the *BMJ*, which is huge. There is a RCGP hot topics course, which is good. Courses take a lot of the legwork away. I didn't go but somebody gave me the notes where they summarise all the research. Four colleagues got into a group and chose a hot topic each to research and bring back to discuss. It cut the work to a quarter.'

Video

'Trainers are not always up to date on what you need to pass. You can waste six months making videos that are useless. I wasn't told you need to have a date and time on each video.

I thought you just videoed what you normally do in daily practice, but they are specific about what they want you to do and ask. My friend said that when any patient came in she would say "Oh, you look really worried" because that is picking up on cues. They want you to share management options, which is hard because doctors are used to saying "Do X, Y and Z and come back to me". You'll fail if you do that. You have to say "Here are the options: we can either do nothing, we could give you antibiotics or we could leave it and review you. What do you want to do?" Older patients don't like that. They say "You're the doctor". If you have a high proportion of refugees who can't speak English, you have difficulty sharing management options.

In one video I had all the cues and asked about family concerns, and it was really good. But the patient had a change in bowel habit and I hadn't done a rectal examination. You'd fail for that. Do a lot more than you think you'll need. Many patients refuse to be videoed or have a boring complaint where you can't get all 15 points in.

You end up following the RCGP pattern. At first I thought this was artificial, but by the end I thought it was useful. But it doesn't work on all the patients. It works if you've got highly intelligent, motivated people to play along.'

■ MRCOG

■ The low-down

The MRCOG (Member of the Royal College of Obstetricians and Gynaecologists) examination is in two parts.

Part 1, held in March and September, is the scientific foundation of obstetrics and gynaecology. It is a prerequisite to entering SpR training, consisting of two MCQ papers, each lasting two hours. Doctors can sit part 1 in their house jobs or as SHOs. There is a 25% pass rate. International postgraduates from countries with comparable training, for example Singapore, may be exempt.

Part 2, also held in March and September, is designed to test theoretical and practical knowledge. Candidates are expected to apply knowledge to management of clinical problems and demonstrate knowledge of practical procedures. It consists of:

- MCQ paper: one two-hour true/false paper
- short-answer questions: five on gynaecology and five on obstetrics
- OSCE.

About 1000 people sit the written component, of which only a quarter pass. Those that pass take an OSCE the following May or November. This has a much higher pass rate, typically between 85–90%.

There are no exemptions for part 2. Initially the College thought that candidates exempted from part 1 might be disadvantaged, but found there is either no difference or people who have exemptions do just as well if not better. Candidates must attempt the part 2 examination within ten years of passing part 1, otherwise they have to pass part 1 again.

■ Cost

Part 1: £235
Part 2: £345

■ Who writes the questions?

Senior college members write questions based on basic scientific principles and decades of clinical experience.

■ Pass mark

MRCOG used to have a fixed pass mark of 75%, but this was abolished as some exams were more difficult. Now a group of examiners goes through every question and works out its difficulty before imposing a pass mark. If an exam is easy the pass mark goes up; if it is harder it goes down.

■ The examiner's view

Elizabeth Owen is Chair of Examiners. 'People fail part 1 if they haven't got enough knowledge of background sciences,' she says. 'Often they haven't learned it at medical school. It is difficult for them to realise that these questions are very relevant, they are very fair, but they are quite scientific. They need to focus on things like "Where are the blood vessels? Where are the nerves? How does the heart work?"

In obs and gynae, life is never true or false, it always depends. It depends whether the woman is five foot tall, whether it's her first baby or her third baby, and on her blood pressure. So we are moving away from true or false questions to using more clinical scenarios and extended matching questions. We have set up an EMQ subcommittee that will spend 18 months developing questions, and then we'll introduce an EMQ element to the written exams.'

So what goes wrong for so many candidates attempting part 2? 'Part 2 is based on UK practice,' says Elizabeth. 'Because 85% of candidates are not from the UK, they don't know a lot of the areas we're talking about. Because they haven't worked here, it is very difficult for them to know about our system. What our College is trying to do is to help people from overseas understand what is expected in the exam by setting up courses throughout the world.'

A lot of candidates struggle with the short essays. Elizabeth suggests: 'Keep up to date, read college guidelines and realise it is a test of use of knowledge. These short answers are not just the writing of an essay on this subject. We ask doctors to justify management of certain cases or debate pros and cons of various treatments. Again, people from overseas often struggle. A lot of people from overseas are not encouraged to question and debate. Didactic teaching prevails and young doctors are told "Don't argue. This is the treatment. This is what I do. This is the drug we use." If you come from a country that has a very didactic teaching style, go on a revision course where they practise short answers and have group discussions. The discussions are about why they answered the way they did and what they should have answered in a different way. In a textbook they don't have the heading "pros and cons of". You have to work that out for yourself.'

■ The candidates' views

Prithi Jain is an SpR at Birmingham Women's Hospital. She did medical training in India and found part 1 very straightforward: 'Part 1 checks medical school knowledge. I'd advise candidates to attempt all questions. People tend to struggle with biochemistry and physiology. I used *Basic Science in Obstetrics and Gynaecology* by Dewhurst, which was very helpful.[10] For part 2, I prepared by working in the UK for a year and a half. It helped a lot as British practice is totally different from what we were doing in a developing country. If you know the system and how to communicate with patients [in the UK], it helps a lot. These things really matter in this exam. People who passed the exam told me not to do more than one course or you can get confused. I went on a revision course at Birmingham Women's Hospital which was fantastic. My colleagues who passed last year went on it and it helped them a lot too. There are some excellent revision books. I'm sure I passed the part 2 written because of Justin Konje's book *Short Essays, MCQs and OSCEs for MRCOG Part 2*.[11] Another thing that I had to get used to was learning to write short answers. You have to write on just one page, so be concise. I recommend spending five minutes planning the question and writing down everything that could be worth a mark. For example, involving the paediatrician, alerting the special care unit, calling the haematologist – and then write your answer. The OSCE is essentially an assessment of what you do in clinic. If you are a good practitioner you shouldn't have any problems.'

Neerja Sharma also trained in India and worked in the Gulf. She chose to work in a clinical attachment in the UK 'because I did part 1 before coming here and that was fine. But part 2 is strongly based on UK practice and you don't get a good idea about that from textbooks. During my clinical attachment I attended the department's meetings and saw how things work. Then when I read around it, everything made much more sense. I have spent all my annual leave for the past two years preparing for the MRCOG. The book which helped me most is *Gynaecology* by Robert Shaw.[12] The new edition is fantastic. For the short answers I used Justin Konje. It is a clear, descriptive book. My consultants in Oman are all members of the College and I went to them for guidance. We talked a lot about protocols, clinical governance and audit. It would help if there was always somebody to answer my questions. You have so much you want to ask and if nobody can help you, you take those doubts to the exam.'

Graham Hutchins is an SpR at Mayday Hospital, South London. 'Don't sit the exam too early,' he warns. 'As a clinician you benefit by doing it when you are part way through your training. I've been on a couple of courses: the Nottingham course and Whipp's Cross course, which is well thought of. I did a lot of work for the written component. That separates people out. There's only a 20% pass rate. I used College guidelines, which are accessible on the web, and if you download these pretty much everything is on there. I haven't picked up a textbook. Remember that OSCEs are what you do day to day.'

■ MRCPsych
■ The low-down

Part 1 of the MRCPsych (Member of the Royal College of Psychiatrists) examination consists of a written and a clinical examination. It is taken after at least 12 months' experience in psychiatry. Before sitting part 2, candidates must have passed, or have been granted exemption from, part 1, and have completed 30 months of full-time post-registration training (or equivalent part-time flexible training) in posts approved by the Royal College of Psychiatrists, by the date of the written papers.

■ Components and requirements

Part 1 has two components:

1 one written paper comprising a mixture of EMQs and individual statement questions (duration: 1 hour 30 minutes)
2 one clinical examination (duration: 1 hour 30 minutes).

Candidates must first pass the written examination before attempting the clinical. To pass, candidates pass the clinical at the same sitting.

Part 2 has four components:

1 two written papers:
   - sciences basic to psychiatry – individual statement questions and EMQs (duration: 1 hour 30 minutes)
   - clinical topics – individual statement questions and EMQs (duration: 1 hour 30 minutes)
2 essay paper – candidates are required to answer one from a choice of three questions covering general and sub-specialty psychiatry. They have to cover the whole life cycle in their essay answers, for example childhood to old age (duration: 1 hour 30 minutes)
3 critical review paper (duration: 1 hour 30 minutes)
4 the clinical examinations:
   - individual patient assessment (duration: 1 hour 30 minutes – 1 hour with the patient followed by 30 minutes with examiners)

- patient management problems (duration: 30 minutes with the examiners). Patient management problems are now standardised. All candidates are asked the same questions on the same day. A brief clinical vignette is followed by a few questions; for example, 'You are asked to assess a 26-year-old in the emergency department who has been brought in by the police, having been found wandering on the streets and taking his clothes off. How would you go about assessing this man?'

■ How much does it cost?

Part 1: £443
Part 2: £525

There is an additional membership fee for successful candidates and an annual retention fee.

■ Who writes the questions?

Members of the Royal College are invited to write EMQs, ISQs and PMPs.

■ The examiner's view

'Part 1 is an assessment of basic skills,' says Anthony Bateman, Deputy Chief Examiner for part 2. 'Candidates should demonstrate a level of skill for someone who has done psychiatry for a year.' He explains that part 2 tries to assess a person's ability to go on to higher training: 'It's an entry exam to SpR training.'

He agrees that many candidates find the critical appraisal paper difficult, but feels it has direct relevance to daily practice: 'One of the recent questions in the critical review paper was "The manager asks how this might inform the organisation of your service". So candidates have to apply results or information to normal clinical work. Many candidates consider that paper to be more tricky than it is. There are no tricks, but candidates look for them and get muddled.'

Anthony explains that when marking patient management problems (PMPs) examiners use several criteria: 'Do candidates approach the scenario appropriately? Do they take safety into account? Do they consider the appropriate diagnostic avenues? Examiners use probes to find out if candidates meet the criteria. The probe might be, what would you advise the nurses when admitting the patient? Or what would you tell the relatives if they asked if their son had got schizophrenia?'

He continues: 'In a patient management problem about a 24-year-old Kurdish refugee, you would have to talk about cultural aspects. You don't need to know masses, but if you don't mention it that would be quite serious. Make sure you don't get a Turkish translator because of the problems between Kurds and Turks. We expect doctors to show some sensitivity to that.'

According to Anthony, many candidates do badly on the essay question: 'Candidates fail because they don't write about the topic they are asked to write about. They write what they know. So if the question says "across the life cycle", you have to put something in about old age and childhood – don't just write about people who are 30. Psychiatrists have to write reports for courts and letters to GPs about complex mental disorders, so that's why the essay paper is there.'

'In the long case, some end up presenting loads of information when actually we want a relevant story, sorted out in the previous hour,' he says. 'We want a mature doctor who puts information together to tell another doctor about it. And the pitfall is that they start to tell it as if they are a medical student. Some omit a physical examination. If a patient is complaining of frequent headaches, the least that they should do is a basic neurological examination.'

Overseas doctors are more likely to fail the long case than UK-trained candidates: 'Overseas doctors may have language difficulties and our exam is language based: clinical interviews, presentations, reading a single statement to see whether it's true or false. We try hard to ensure that statements don't have a nuance that only native English speakers would understand. The other aspect overseas doctors find difficult is the clinical. Often their knowledge is excellent, but they might not have had enough practice within our system.'

Many candidates are nervous about patients who may be uncooperative in the long case. 'If anything untoward happens like the patient walks out, that is noted by the people on the ground and the examiner has that information,' says Anthony. 'So we try to ensure people are not disadvantaged by a more problematic case.'

He feels revision courses are 'probably OK for knowledge but not for skills. Part 2 is trying to assess a practising psychiatrist after two and a half to three years' training. It is not trying to assess someone who's mugged everything up in two months.' In his opinion, 'Small working groups of people taking the exam are essential, so that they learn together, discuss topics and actually present cases with a senior person and practise some patient management problems. Do critical appraisal through an evidence-based journal club.'

What are the examiners looking for? 'A safe, sensitive, knowledgeable psych-iatrist who is suitable to go through to higher training,' says Anthony. 'They must have a high level of knowledge on a wide range of areas. They must have a good level of pharmacology and how drugs interact. They also must have a basic level of psychological treatments. They need to know some basic neurology, differentiating early dementia in 50-year-olds from depression.'

■ The candidates' views

Stephanie Young is an SpR at Guy's and St Thomas' Hospital, London. She spends a special interest session each week preparing candidates for MRCPsych. 'I used a combination of private study and group study,' she says, 'and for the clinical I did a lot of practice presentations to SpRs and consultants.' Stephanie failed part 1 at her first attempt, but learned 'it wasn't because I hadn't studied enough, but because of poor technique. It isn't the end of the world to fail. I'd advise others who fail not to take it personally. I did change strategy though and my revision became more exam focused. I went on several MRCPsych courses. I like the superego café website.' She also advises against using too many textbooks. 'For OSCEs,' she continues, 'read through the Royal College leaflets for hints on how to explain mental illnesses in lay terms. And try mind mapping, developed by Tony Buzan.'[13]

'For part 1, I got organised eight weeks before the exam,' says Paul Wheelan, SHO at South London and Maudsley NHS Trust. 'I went through thousands of MCQs and from there went to textbooks and then looked up the answers.' Paul then went on the NB course, which he likes as he found it 'orientated towards the exam'. For the part 1 clinical, Paul presented 20 cases in exam style to different consultants. 'One of the consultants videotaped me presenting cases about ten times,' he recalls. 'It was superb. It was anxiety provoking so I'd habituated by the time the clinical exam came along. When I watched the videos I noticed how I slouched and so I held my shoulders back. I also didn't think I made enough eye contact. Those things are important and I would recommend videoing. You notice a lot more about your technique, like certain catchphrases you need to eradicate.'

Paul studied hard for four months prior to the part 2 written: 'I did ISQs, EMQs, essays. I went on the Guildford course six months before the exam because I knew it would take time to learn how to write an essay and it required a lot of book learning.' Like Stephanie, he found the critical appraisal paper particularly difficult: 'I got that book *Critical Appraisal for Psychiatrists*.[14] It was like reading Russian. I started reading it six months before the exam. I read it twice from cover to cover just to get it into my head.' When it came to part 2 clinicals, Paul presented to ten different consultants and was videoed again. 'I recommend going to lots of different consultants,' he says. 'Part 2 examiners are the most helpful people to present to. They taught me to present patients in the way I felt most comfortable.'

■ MRCPCH and DCH

■ The low-down

The Royal College of Paediatrics and Child Health runs two examinations: the MRCPCH, required for entry into higher specialist training, and the Diploma of Child Health (DCH). The DCH is designed primarily for GPs but is also suitable for any doctor involved in looking after children, for example child psychiatry or ENT surgery. The DCH is not a requirement but an additional qualification.

Part 1a is written and consists of MCQs, best of five and EMQs. It is on general aspects of child health and is common to those taking MRCPCH and DCH. Candidates sitting DCH go on to a separate clinical exam.

Part 1b is similar: MCQs, best of five and EMQs on the scientific basis of paediatrics and extended knowledge.

Part 2 consists of written and clinical exams. There are two papers with best of five or EMQs about case histories, data interpretation and photographic material. From October 2004 the clinical is going to be a multi-station exam. There will be two communication stations, one history taking and management planning station, and one video station with six to eight videos and six clinical short cases. The short cases will include child development, examination of the cardiovascular system, a neurology and neurodisability case, and three others. Most stations will be nine minutes each. History taking and videos are double stations.

■ How much does it cost?

Part 1a: £135
For those going on to DCH clinical after Part 1a: £210
An extra £75 for a DCH certificate and to be able to use the letters DCH after your name
Part 1b: £135
Part 2 written: £280
Part 2 clinical: £400

The prices are only applicable for those sitting the exam in the UK. Fees vary in other countries.

■ Who writes the questions?

A panel of paediatricians recruited by the Royal College.

■ Pass mark

At the time of writing the College was unable to tell us what the pass marks for the new-style exam would be 'because the structure is going to be new'. They did say the pass mark would vary with each exam and 'DCH is going to have a higher pass mark. It is a voluntary exam and if one was going to have a 20% pass mark, everyone would say that is not appropriate. While clearly people have to do a lot of preparation and work for it, getting a national training number is a bigger hurdle.'

■ The examiner's view

'Would you like this person to be your SpR tomorrow? That's the criteria we use for this exam,' says Tom Lissauer, Officer for Examinations at the Royal College of Paediatrics and Child Health. 'In our exam a lot is about dealing with emergencies because that is the most important thing we require of a newly appointed SpR.'

Before the new-style clinicals, examiners will see the children and agree what they expect candidates to achieve. Tom explains: 'We are looking for candidates to demonstrate they are used to handling parents and children. If children are not happy, we are looking for candidates being able to handle that.'

Tom feels the main reason for failure is lack of experience: 'There is a temptation for people to take the exam too early. Everybody is so keen to progress that they just have a go and see what it's like. That is not the wisest way.'

The College doesn't recommend any books or revision material other than 'our past papers and stuff on the web'.

'One problem,' says Tom, 'is people spend too much time learning how to take the exam and not enough time going back to the basics of knowledge and experience. If people think they are going to pass the exam by practising millions of multiple-choice questions, that is a poor way of preparing.'

■ The candidate's view

'For part 1, do lots of practice questions, which you can get from books,' advises Meena Patel, SHO at Great Ormond Street, London. She did part 1 in her first year of SHO training and part 2 in her second year, passing both first time. The College has sample papers, which Meena used as the basis of her revision rather than using books first: 'I did lots of questions using Pastest books. I particularly like *Essential Revision Notes for Paediatrics* by Beattie.[15] And go on courses. I went on a Pastest as they give you a huge range of questions.'

'It's not a pleasant thing,' says Meena, reminiscing about part 2. 'Because this is a new style of exam, we weren't sure what to expect. It was quite stressful. The main advice everybody gave me for the written is to do lots of questions as you are revising, then look at books, rather than the other way round. The more questions you do, the more likely you are to come across cases that will come up.'

There are few revision books available that focus on the new part 2. Meena recommends 'the Churchill Livingstone series: they've got good data books; they've got picture books. A great book I used was *Paediatric Grey Cases for the MRCPCH.*'[16]

She used these books to look up and learn answers to questions rather than trying to read them: 'Everyone does different things but a lot of people advised me to do that.' The same questions come up year after year so the more you see, the more you recognise. That is one of the most useful things.'

'With the clinicals learning is different,' says Meena. 'Do lots of practice with registrars grilling you with viva questions, so when examiners do the same you're not thrown.' She adds: 'Put a bad case behind you and don't let it fluff you. If you get flustered you are at a disadvantage for your next short case or OSCE station.'

Meena suggests candidates think carefully about when to do the exam: 'Do part 1 early, but part 2 needs clinical experience. In certain jobs like neonates, it is difficult to find patients suitable for exam practice. Busy jobs make it difficult to study.'

■ MRCPath
■ The low-down

The MRCPath (Member of the Royal College of Pathologists) examination differs for each specialist, i.e. haematologists, immunologists, histopathologists, forensic pathologists, biochemists and molecular geneticists; there is a whole portfolio of examinations for different subspecialties. MRCPath is unique among membership examinations as it is also taken by non-medics, including vets and toxicologists. For histopathology and immunology exams, there are typically only two or three candidates at each sitting.

Detailed examination regulations and guidelines for all the different MRCPath exams can be found on the Royal College website: www.rcpath.org.

Although MRCPath is taken at the end of specialist training, it isn't an exit exam because the Royal College considers the Certificate of Completion of Specialist Training (CCST) to be the exit qualification. Part 1 is usually taken after one to three years of higher specialist training. It is a test of knowledge, understanding and practical aspects. Candidates are usually just into SpR level. Part 2 is taken after a minimum of four years' training. Many of the MRCPath exams contain objective structured pathology examinations (OSPEs). Most also contain a clinical component.

■ How much does it cost?

Part 1: all specialties (except histopathology, new medical microbiology and virology)
Part 1 written: £250
Part 1 practical and oral: £250

Part 2: all specialties (except histopathology, new medical microbiology and virology)
Part 2 practical or oral: £275

Parts 1 and 2 histopathology (and part 2 related subspecialties)
Part 1 written: £250
Part 2 practical: £525

Parts 1 and 2 new medical microbiology
Part 1 multiple-choice question: £250
Part 2 written: £250
Part 2 practical and oral: £275

■ Pass rate

The Royal College told us that they 'don't have the IT support' to know the exact pass rate, but estimate it at around 80%.

■ The examiner's view

'We are unique in being the only multi-professional College,' says Clair du Boulay, Chair of the Examinations Committee, 'and our exams reflect that. MRCPath isn't an exam that most people fail as candidates are usually well prepared. Our exam isn't a screening exam, but a test of competencies towards the end of training. We expect most people to pass. It is criterion referenced. We don't have a set percentage to fail.'

Clair explains that people who fail tend to be those who haven't been in proper training programmes. 'Others fail because they are no good,' she continues. 'Some don't put in the time and effort. The majority of people who fail don't know their stuff. They make mistakes diagnosing and would be dangerous. I would be up for failing someone who was a non-communicator, but so far we only fail people who don't know enough.'

Clair feels the exams are designed to test knowledge, skills, aptitude, attitudes and communication. 'For example, a histopathologist will have to do an autopsy as part of their part 2,' she says. The College has been looking at ways of making examination of the autopsy more objective and are introducing a scenario-based exam where a pathologist might be asked to explain, for example, why they are doing an autopsy on someone's baby to a simulated relative. 'Being able to communicate with a family is important,' believes Clair. 'Recent issues with autopsies have highlighted that we need to examine histopathologists' communication skills.'

She is keen to stress MRCPath is 'not just testing pathology but also professional practice. If a candidate is rigid and not prepared to say they don't know, we feel worried about them. We don't recommend people put themselves forward unless they are in a proper training programme in the UK or overseas. They need to have proper supervision that prepares them for the exam.'

Some of those who have failed the exam include overseas doctors who have been working as professors in their home countries. 'We recommend doctors from overseas work in a UK training programme for a short time before sitting the exam,' says Clair. 'There are enormous cultural differences in how people are taught. They come here and see that it is OK to ask a question. That's an advantage, as in a viva they will be able to have a debate.'

She explains a College dilemma: 'We often wonder if the exam should be tailor-made for the UK and test British diseases. But is it fair for someone who has worked in Africa to be tested on essentially UK health problems? Diseases are different in different parts of the world, and our view is that our examinations are really to test people in the UK.'

According to Clair, it is important for candidates to 'demonstrate they have taken into account a range of differential diagnoses. We are not looking for right and wrong. We are looking for safe practice and for doctors to say when they don't know. That's what patients need.'

■ The candidate's view

'A lot of people struggle to get part 1,' says Daniel Scott, a consultant histopathologist at Harrogate District Hospital. 'People look at it as a mountain of knowledge – hundreds of papers, hundreds of articles – thinking "Oh my God, where do I start?".' Daniel's solution was 'a problem-orientated approach. Some people read every article published over the last two years, thinking they're bound to come up because they are trendy and new. That is a failing attitude because it is not focused. I made a list of all the topics that were going to be covered and for each I read one or two articles, sometimes from a textbook, sometimes from a journal.' Daniel particularly liked Lowe and Underwood's *Recent Advances in Histopathology*,[17] Kirkham's *Progress in Pathology*[18] and Herrington's *Current Diagnostic Pathology*.[19] For general articles, he recommends *Robbins' Pathological Basis of Disease*.[20]

He then spent four months producing revision material: 'Some people claim to have read 1000-page textbooks twice, and I either don't believe them or they have amazing ability to concentrate and read a book. Remember that no examiner will expect you to write a four-page essay on an incredibly rare disease. Examiners aren't that unrealistic. A lot of my work was putting my base together: photo-copying articles and putting them in four lever arch files. And for the last month I hardly looked at a book but read those lever arch files three or four times.'

'I think a lot of people come unstuck on the questions of practice in pathology,' says Daniel.' These questions try to establish whether people have practical experience in seeing how things work. It is NHS focused and you get questioned on things like audit, management scenarios and quality control – all that sort of stuff. In my view those questions are the easiest. There is no right or wrong answer – how would you improve the error rate in pathology, for example. But people avoid them and answer some question on an obscure disease that they don't really know anything about. For the obscure you have got to know facts. If you don't, you've had it. But if you've got knowledge of NHS systems and common sense, they have to give you marks. Exams are about harvesting marks, aren't they?'

Daniel elaborates on how important it is to think about marks. 'Because of closed marking you can't afford to fail one part of the exam,' he warns. 'They are marked out of ten. Three is fail; four is a pass and five a good pass. You've got to average 16 for the four passes. If you get three that means that you have to make it up with a five, and it is virtually impossible to get a five. A lot of people look at a question and think "that's my weak answer and I won't invest much time on it", but you've got to be able to answer four questions.'

'Not many people fail on autopsies,' says Daniel. 'But what people do trip up on is that they don't present themselves in a professional manner. It's your first physical exposure to the examiner, your chance to get that examiner confident in you. You know what you're doing, you're capable, you're competent and you know you've got some interpersonal skills and can present your findings formally.

Exams are full of myths. Autopsy has special techniques, done very occasionally to specific parts of the body – like the spinal column or middle ear – and people get really hung up about these. There are stories about people being asked to do these things, but I don't know anyone who was asked to do anything pretty difficult. It's there to test your training. You are much more likely to be asked about dealing with a coroner and death certification.'

Daniel recommends candidates find someone else who is doing the exam: 'You can enthuse each other and rub off each other. With double-headed microscopes you can look at the same thing. One puts a slide in and tests the other one. It's a very good way of learning, much more dynamic and less tedious than doing it on your own. People have weak points and strong points. I learned a lot from the person I worked with and he learned a lot from me.'

■ FRCA

■ The low-down

The FRCA (Fellow of the Royal College of Anaesthetists) examination is in two parts, the primary and the final (also called fellowship). Primary FRCA can be taken after one year in an approved SHO post.

■ Primary FRCA

There are four sections:

1 90 MCQs of three hours' duration, with approximately 30 questions in pharmacology, 30 questions in physiology and biochemistry, and 30 questions in physics and clinical measurement

2 An OSCE of approximately 1 hour 40 minutes, currently comprising 16 stations covering resuscitation, technical skills, anatomy, history taking, physical examination, communication skills, interpretation of ECG, X-ray and interpreting investigation results, statistics, anaesthetic equipment, monitoring equipment, measuring equipment and anaesthetic hazards
3 viva 1 – a 30-minute structured viva voce comprising 15 minutes in pharmacology and 15 minutes in physiology and biochemistry
4 viva 2 – a 30 minute structured viva voce comprising 15 minutes in physics, clinical measurement, equipment and safety, and 15 minutes on clinical topics (including a critical incident).

Doctors with primary FRCA are eligible to apply for SpR jobs. They work between one to two years before sitting the final FRCA. The College strongly recommends candidates should only sit the final FRCA after a minimum of six months in a LAT, FTTA or SpR post. Doctors usually take the final as a second-year SpR. It is the entry requirement for SpR training years three, four and five.

■ Final FRCA

There are four sections:

1 90 MCQs, again lasting three hours, comprising approximately 20 questions in medicine and surgery; 40 questions in anaesthesia and pain management, including applied basic sciences (mainly pharmacology and physiology); ten questions in clinical measurement and 20 questions in intensive therapy
2 short-answer question (SAQ) paper with 12 compulsory questions – three hours on the principles and practice of clinical anaesthesia
3 viva 1 – 50 minutes on clinical anaesthesia. A structured viva voce comprising ten minutes to view clinical material, 20 minutes of questions on the material and 20 minutes of questions on unrelated clinical anaesthesia
4 viva 2 – 30 minutes of clinical science. A structured viva voce on application of basic science to anaesthesia, intensive therapy and pain management.

■ How much does it cost?

Primary: £505
Final: £605

Both examinations are increasing by £10 from September 2004.

■ Who writes the questions?

A panel of experts draws on academic and clinical experience.

■ Pass rate

The pass rate for the last exam was 48%. For the primary exam it is usually between 45–50%.

■ The examiner's view

Andrew Mortimer is Chair of the Examinations Committee of the Royal College of Anaesthetists' overseas and primary and final FRCA examinations. He agrees with Martin's final comment: 'In our specialty if you make a misjudgment, you kill the patient; and for any candidate that makes a suggestion that is profoundly wrong, it's an outright fail. Even if they've passed everything else, patient safety is our main goal. So we look for judgement. Candidates can know all the facts, but can they make decisions and apply them quickly? They are given clinical scenarios to deal with and asked how they would proceed. There is not one correct answer, there are probably several, but we are testing reasoning and the understanding.'

The Royal College of Anaesthetists provides mandatory examination counselling. Andrew elaborates: 'If you fail the primary twice, you have to undergo mandatory guidance with two experienced examiners and ideally your college tutor. All the exam papers you have failed are available for you to see what you are doing wrong.'

'We don't have any quotas. There are always people who will underperform. In the final exam the pass mark is between 50–55%, which is what you'd expect. Most people have got it after three attempts. Knowledge, skills and attitudes are our three big headings. Attend all the courses made available for you: College regional courses, lectures and those run by various enterprising people as well.'

Andrew agrees that doctors from overseas find the exam harder: 'It's a personal observation, but there are cultural differences and attitudes towards patients. If you come from certain countries, patients can be like lumps of meat, while here we are more lovey-dovey. We have a greater culture of involving patients. In the exam we have communication stations and candidates are observed explaining things to patients. Doctors taught in a more didactic way should practise in front of observing consultants.'

The bottom line?
'I want to know that the guys and gals sitting the exam can give me an anaesthetic and not kill me in the process.'

■ The candidates' views

'I won't bother resitting if I fail,' says Mark Wilson, who passed all parts of the MRCS first time round before subjecting himself to the FRCA. He passed the primary MCQs at his first attempt and is now studying for the OSCEs and vivas. 'Revise hard,' he says. This may be easier said than done, and Mark admits that the hardest part of the FRCA is 'finding the time to revise'. He found the website www.frca.co.uk useful.

Martin Ruth is a consultant anaesthetist with the Royal Air Force in Edinburgh. 'I took my exams more frequently than I would have liked to,' he recalls. 'If I'd knuckled down for six months it wouldn't have been such a trauma, but I brought failure upon myself.'

Martin was told 'in no uncertain terms how difficult it would be and I knuckled down, did the work and fell at the last hurdle in one of the vivas. I got taken to bits. It was one of those things: he saw me floundering and he went in for the kill.'

'You have to devote time and effort,' says Martin. 'I was a bit half-hearted. It is unlikely that you will fail the exams unless you really aren't applying yourself. I can say that because I failed exams in university and then postgraduate exams, and it was because I didn't do the work. Having other people doing the exam with you is always a big help – meetings and little clubs do help.'

Martin attended a three-week course at the College for the final part, which he found very helpful. He also recommends finding somewhere quiet to study: 'The library was the best place for me. If I went home I'd never do any work. You find in the months preceding there will be a review article or editorial that will come up as one of the questions. Both the *British Journal of Anaesthesia* (*BJA*) and *Anaesthesia* should form part of your study programme. The Association of Anaesthetists produces little booklets, which are useful for topics such as treating Jehovah's Witnesses. You'd be a fool not to expect that one because it deals with blood issues.'

He also used CD-ROMs of vivas and MCQs and found them 'bloody difficult, but they weren't far off the mark. With MCQs you have to do as many as possible. It doesn't matter where they are from. Just get your hands on them.'

'If you mention something out of the blue then that is fair game to be talked about. Don't put yourself in it. If they grab onto it and you don't know what you're talking about,' warns Martin, 'and if you make a comment that is downright dangerous or miss something like forgetting to give an asthmatic oxygen, these are cardinal sins and will fail you.'

■ MFPH

■ The low-down

The MFPH (Membership of the Faculty of Public Health) examination consists of the diploma and part 1, and part 2. Passing the diploma and part 1 examination leads to Diplomate Membership, and passing part 2 leads to full Membership of the Faculty of Public Health. The diploma and part 1 test knowledge and understanding of the scientific basis of public health. They are made up of the following written components:

1 Paper 1 (four hours) – the so-called 'knowledge paper'. There are ten compulsory short-answer questions on core sciences of public health. Most questions will be prefaced by 'write short notes on'. Paper 1 is in two sections:
   • section A (2.5 hours). Six questions covering:
     – research methods, including epidemiology, statistical methods, and other methods including qualitative research methods
     – disease prevention and health promotion
     – health information

- section B (1.5 hours). Four questions covering:
  - medical sociology, social policy and health economics
  - organisation and management of healthcare.
2 Paper 2 (4 hours) – the so-called 'skills paper'. This paper tests public health skills. It is also in two sections:
  - section A (2.5 hours). Critical appraisal and commentary based on an article from a journal and application to a specific public health problem. The second half of the question may be phrased in general terms and allow candidates to give examples from different contexts
  - section B (1.5 hours). Candidates have to synthesise a range of materials and produce a summary, policy or other document aimed at a particular target individual or group. Data manipulation and interpretation may form part of this.

Part 2 is designed to test application of knowledge, skills and attitudes to public health. It has two components:

1 *written submission* – candidates produce between two and four reports demonstrating four key competencies for practice, chosen by members of the Faculty. They are critical literary review, health needs assessment, information for planning health services and evaluation of the effectiveness of healthcare and health services. Taken together, the word count for the whole submission (covering all four competencies) must not exceed 20 000 words.
2 *oral examination* – candidates are invited to summarise their written submission and are then questioned on specific aspects of it. The second part of the oral exam is spent discussing issues in public health.

■ How much does it cost?

Part 1: £450
Part 2: £506

■ Who writes the questions?

The questions are set by the Faculty examiners. There is an annual exam-setting meeting every September to choose papers for the following year. In the last couple of years the Faculty has started to develop a question bank and now draws some questions from the bank. A bank of general oral questions is available online at: www.fphm.org.uk/Exams/PartII/The_General_Oral_Question_Bank.shtml

■ What is the pass rate?

The pass rate is 60% at each sitting.

■ The examiners' views

'People lack clarity,' says Professor Brian McLoskey, Chief Examiner for Part 2 Membership of the Faculty of Public Health. 'We advise them to ensure that their reports are directed towards the competency. A good piece doesn't necessarily demonstrate the competency that you are trying to get. Being clear about it in writing and in the drawing up of conclusions and action plans is essential.

Make sure that you stay focused on the competency you are trying to deliver. Put it away and come back and read it again. You get so wrapped up in writing it, you get mixed up at the beginning and the end. Get somebody else to read it through who can give you advice on whether it makes sense or not. Do conclusions flow naturally from the results? If you put it away and come back to it later, you see where the typos are and the logic fails.'

'Each person in training in public health will have a service and academic supervisor allocated,' explains Brian. 'They will give guidance both in choice of the projects and writing up. We also produce guidance made from feedback to candidates going back five years – good and bad points – and there is the opportunity to sit down and talk to one of the examiners about any project work. Most deaneries also run general question sessions based on any range of topics related to public health and mock vivas.'

Reports can be submitted on three occasions every year. What happens to them? 'The report goes out to two examiners who mark it independently,' explains Brian. 'Then they are told who the other marker is and exchange notes and agree a common mark. You are invited to London for an examination on it. The two examiners plus one observer will ask you questions: clarification or things they disagree with. The grades you can get on your submissions are a provisional pass, provisional fail and, depending on your oral, pass or fail. You could pass two reports and bank them and fail the other two. So you'd only have to retake the competencies you'd failed.'

Brian also explains there are changes in the pipeline: 'In about three years we will have moved to an electronic computer-based, simulation-based model.'

'We can spot when one examiner is being unduly influenced by another,' says Stephen George, chief examiner for part 1 and a reader in public health at the University of Southampton. 'Each examiner marks all papers in their section and sends their unconferred marks to the Faculty; then they talk between themselves and agree a mark for each candidate.'

Stephen says that although 'not everyone has to be a statistical genius, candidates need an element of numeracy.' He continues: 'We would much rather have people who say "I don't know what this statistical test is; I'll have to go and look it up" than people who make wild guesses.' He also outlines the most common reasons for failure: 'One is extensive variability: good at one bit of the exam and rotten at another. Some people are never going to be numerate and you can speculate whether you can ever train them. I'm not sure one can. One can improve people who've got a basic level, but there are some people who will never see numbers. It's a very professional exam; it's about competency in the things we are asking people to do. We won't usually ask people to calculate complement intervals in an exam, but we will ask them to calculate the relative risks.'

■ The candidate's view

'You fail part 1 if you don't answer all the questions,' says Ash Paul, an SpR working for the National Public Health Service for Wales. Ash revised by 'getting hold of past questions and writing out answers within an allocated time span.' His textbooks of choice for part 1: 'One is written by the present Chief Medical Officer of England, and was originally started by his dad: *Essential Public Health Medicine* by Donaldson and Donaldson.[21] The other helpful book is *The Oxford Handbook of Public Health Practice* by David Pencheon.'[22]

Ash explains how the competencies for part 2 can be written: 'One of my reports had three competencies and another had one. But the danger in having a three-in-one is that if you fail one of the competencies, the whole project fails. You have to submit all three competencies again.'

His first project, which gained him three competencies, was a review and reconfiguration of maternity units in North-West Wales: 'The problem was that there were three GP-led maternity units and the GPs came along and said "We aren't going to be supplying services to these hospitals any more". These hospitals are in the depths of rural North Wales. So the health authority had to come up with a solution. My director of public health asked me to review the entire service and come up with an alternative solution. I led on the project, taking advice from my director at regular intervals, and the three competencies were answered by a critical examination of the literature.' Ash looked especially at the following questions: 'Are new ways of organising maternity services associated with different clinical outcomes? Are they safe? What are the good and bad points of these research articles?'

'The hardest part is the needs assessment,' he says of the competencies. 'Not only counting numbers, but taking all the stakeholders – including service users – into account. I had to devise a questionnaire survey for pregnant women who had delivered in GP units to find out their views: "If the hospital closed down, would you be happy to use a consultant-led unit in Bangor, 60 miles away, or a midwife-led unit here?".'

Ash has helpful suggestions for candidates who are asked to resubmit their work: 'They have to give you the specific points to work on. Answer each point. It could mean doing extra pieces of work.' One of his colleagues, for instance, was told she hadn't taken account of the views of users. He suggests: 'Go to the website and you'll see examiners have come up with a series of questions in each competency that they expect the examinee to have answered in their project.'

Finally, he raves about 'a very good practical course for the oral, run by Dr Jean Richards, a part 2 examiner. She is exceedingly good. She gives you mock vivas, tells you whether you've written rubbish and asks critical questions. She will tell you about using a proper structure.'

■ References

1 *The IELTS Handbook* can be downloaded for free from www.ielts.org/library/handbook_2003.pdf

2 Coales U (2002) *PLAB: 1000 extended matching questions.* Royal Society of Medicine Press Ltd, London.

3 Kroker P (2002) *PLAB Part 1 EMQ Pocket Book: book 3.* Pastest Books, Cheshire.

4 Beynon H (1991) *The Complete MRCP Part 1: MCQs.* Churchill Livingstone, Edinburgh.

5 Sharma S (2000) *Rapid Review of Clinical Medicine.* Manson Publishing Ltd, London.

6 Ryder (1998) *An Aid to the MRCP Short Cases.* Blackwell Science, Oxford.

7 Baliga R (2002) *250 Cases in Clinical Medicine (MRCP Study Guides)*. Saunders, Oxford.

8 Warrell D, Cox T, Firth J, Benz EJ (2003) *Oxford Textbook of Medicine*. Oxford University Press, Oxford.

9 Lowe D (2001) *General Pathology Vivas*. Greenwich Medical Media Ltd, London.

10 Dewhurst CJ (ed) (1992) *Basic Science in Obstetrics and Gynaecology*. Churchill Livingstone, Edinburgh.

11 Konje J (2003) *Short Essays, MCQs and OSCEs for MRCOG Part 2*. Hodder Arnold, London.

12 Shaw RW (ed) (2002) *Gynaecology*. Churchill Livingstone, London.

13 Buzan T (2003) *How to Mind Map: make the most of your mind and learn how to create, organise and plan.* HarperCollins, London.

14 Lawrie SM, McIntosh AM and Rao S (2000) *Critical Appraisal for Psychiatrists.* Churchill Livingstone, London.

15 Beattie RM (2002) *Essential Revision Notes for Paediatrics*. Pastest Books, Cheshire.

16 Fenton A and Eastham EJ (2001) *Paediatric Grey Cases for the MRCPCH*. Churchill Livingstone, London.

17 Lowe D and Underwood JCE (2001) *Recent Advances in Histopathology*. Churchill Livingstone, London.

18 Kirkham N (2003) *Progress in Pathology*. Greenwich Medical Media Ltd, London.

19 Herrington CS and McGee JO'D (eds) (1993) *Diagnostic Molecular Pathology: a practical approach*. Oxford University Press, Oxford.

20 Cotran RS, Kumar V and Robbins SL (1994) *Robbins' Pathological Basis of Disease*. Saunders, Oxford.

21 Donaldson LJ and Donaldson RJ (2000) *Essential Public Health Medicine*. Petroc Press, Newbury.

22 Pencheon D (ed) (2001) *The Oxford Handbook of Public Health Practice*. Oxford University Press, Oxford.

■ Further reading

Anderson M and Jankowski J (2001) Higher research degrees: making the right choice. *BMJ*. **322**: A2.

Campbell S and Lees C (2000) *Obstetrics by Ten Teachers* (17e). Hodder Arnold, London.

Clayton SG (2004) *Gynaecology by Ten Teachers*. Arnold, London.

Collier J, Longmore M and Scally P (2003) *Oxford Handbook of Clinical Specialties*. Oxford University Press, Oxford.

Ellis H and Calne RY (2003) *Lecture Notes on General Surgery*. Blackwell Science, Oxford.

Kumar PJ and Clark ML (2002) *Clinical Medicine*. Saunders, Oxford.

Lloyd-Williams M (2002) Working full time while studying for a higher degree. *BMJ*. **324**: S68.

Montgomery H, Goldsack N, Marshall R *et al.* (2003) *My First MRCP Book*. REMEDICA Publishing Ltd, London.

CHAPTER 7

Hard times

It was the best of times, it was the worst of times, it was the age of
wisdom, it was the age of foolishness, it was the epoch of belief, it was
the epoch of incredulity, it was the season of light, it was the season of
darkness, it was the spring of hope, it was the winter of despair.

Charles Dickens, author, 1812–1870

■ Hard times

What keeps me going is hope. I believe in fate and destiny. But you have
to do your bit, and if you believe in what you do and if you do everything
you can, then eventually you will get there. You can't stay at home and
wait. Do things to make it happen. But if after you have done your best it
doesn't work out, then it's not in your destiny. Don't kill yourself over it.

Otmane El Mezoued, refugee doctor from Algeria

When you live abroad you go through stages. The first stage is that everything is very novel, so you have a honeymoon period where everything is
interesting. The second stage is a homesickness period: you're nostalgic,
everything back home is better and you're struggling with people and
relationships. The third is that you think some things are better there and
some things are better here, and the fourth stage is no difference: people
are people once you get to know them. The same things hurt them and
give them joy.

Zerrin Atakan from Turkey, Lead Consultant, National Psychosis Unit

An international doctor's life is sometimes hard, often unfair. Bureaucratic regulations, baffling systems, the great British reserve and grey skies quash the spirit
of even the keenest and most enthusiastic. A failed exam, bout of flu or racist insult
can make you feel like giving up and getting out. This chapter gives practical
advice on what to do when life gets difficult and points you towards sources of
help.

The title of this chapter, 'Hard times', is taken from a novel by Charles Dickens.
The quote below the title comes from another Dickens masterpiece, *A Tale of Two
Cities*: a story about love and loyalty set in Paris and London at the time of
the French Revolution. Although written in 1859, we believe the issues he raises
have relevance for international doctors today. Divided loyalties, homesickness,
estrangement in a foreign country and two suitors competing for a doctor's

daughter make a compelling tale. Dickens' quotation is particularly apposite as he wrote *A Tale of Two Cities* during the most difficult period of his adult life. It remains one of his most popular books. During hard times we often learn and achieve great things.

■ Failing exams

> Generally it is our failures that civilise us. Triumph confirms us in our habits.
>   Clive James (1939–), Australian writer and broadcaster

> You look at people that have graduated overseas and you find they have a much lower pass rate. That's not discrimination. It's the fact that the expectation is that the doctor will be suitable for an English patient, so all of that is part of the culturisation that somebody coming to this country needs to undertake.
>   Professor Michael Cormi, British GP

Failure hurts, let no one tell you otherwise. Few pains equal that of scrolling through a list of people who have passed a membership exam that you have taken, only to discover your name is not there. Feelings of panic may follow – confusion, anger, disbelief (surely there has been a mistake) – before the news sinks in. Others have passed and can move on; you can't. Others will be out celebrating while you will be at home licking your wounds. Then there is the self-reproach: feeling you have let the side down – family, friends and tutors; that you might just have got through had you put in a little more effort and application. You might feel angry with yourself for daring to have thought you were in with a chance. Then there is the public knowledge of your failure – the pleasure it will give to the people who dislike you.

Disappointing though these setbacks are, most people have tripped up in their medical careers at one time or other. In the long run, not passing PLAB part 2 first time round may prove only to be a minor blip rather than the major calamity it seems at the time.

Don't panic if you fail:

- IELTS
- PLAB
- postgraduate examinations.

Many doctors from the UK and abroad sit exams more than once before passing. Don't worry if you are one of them. Failure is a very common experience and one that feels especially unfair if you have worked hard, studied for long hours and are then unsuccessful. When you fail an exam you will feel like giving up. You may also feel upset, cheated, angry, exhausted, bitter, homesick and worried about the future.

■ Tips for surviving failure

1 Remember that failing exams doesn't mean you have failed at life. Put it in perspective.

2 Ask for feedback. You may have to pay for written feedback. It can help you structure your next phase of revision as you will see you are not bad at all parts of the exam.
3 Surround yourself with helpful people: your study group, friends, tutors and consultants will help you if you ask them.
4 Many people fail because of poor technique. Could this apply to you? You may not need to learn a lot more facts, but instead concentrate on applying facts and focus on parts of the exam you struggled with.

■ Racism

There is tremendous prejudice against overseas doctors. They don't mind them doing junior work, but when it comes to consultant level it becomes much more difficult. It is only in the Cinderella specialties that there are really large numbers of consultants from ethnic minorities. If you come here as a surgeon and think 'I'll be a consultant surgeon in England', I think your chances are about nil. If you come as a psychogeriatrician, you have a good chance of getting a consultant job.

Professor Michael Cormi, British GP

You always have to prove you are better than local graduates to get noticed.
Yong Lok Ong, consultant old age psychiatrist from Singapore and
Overseas Doctors Dean, London Deanery

I've been called Paki a few times.
Samja Mishra, SHO in ophthalmology from India

On paper, all jobs are advertised and appointed with regard to *equal opportunities policy*. This means that there must be no discrimination with regard to sex, colour, race, nationality, disability and ethnic origin.

It is a sad fact of life that racism exists. Racism has been defined as 'conduct or words or practices which disadvantage or advantage people because of their colour, culture or ethnic origin'.[1] Discrimination on grounds of race and colour exists in UK medicine as elsewhere in society. In institutional racism there is a belief that whites are 'better' than other ethnic groups, who should therefore be subordinate. What is clear is that popular specialties which are oversubscribed tend to be full of UK-trained graduates, while the so-called Cinderella specialties are more willing to employ international doctors.

Some ground-breaking research was conducted by Aneez Esmail and Sam Everington in 1993.[2] They found significant evidence that applicants with Asian surnames were less likely to obtain a first SHO post than applicants with Anglo-Saxon surnames, despite identical CVs. A follow-up study in 1997 showed only slight improvement and there was still a marked difference between the proportion of white (52%) and Asian applicants (36%) being shortlisted.[3]

Other studies by the same authors demonstrated that white consultants are three times more likely to receive merit awards[4] and Asian doctors are six times more likely to be disciplined by the GMC.[5]

Whether you wish to enter into a specialty known to be welcoming to international doctors, or to try and make it in one of the more popular ones, is a personal matter. It should be noted that Professor Cormi's remarks at the start of this section are made by somebody who has been helpful to overseas and refugee doctors.

> Find people who will listen to you and advise you and find people to tackle it. As medical director, I wrote reprimand letters to consultants who made racist comments to junior doctors. It changed their behaviour but not their personality. Make sure there is nothing wrong with what you are doing. We can't change the world but we can change ourselves. I have seen people using the race card for all the problems in the world.
>
> Umesh Prabhu, consultant paediatrician from India

■ Refugee doctors

> When I came to the UK I did small jobs because I couldn't communicate. I worked as a cleaner. I was so good at it I became a supervisor cleaner. You can be a supervisor cleaner without English. I didn't feel bad but thought 'I have to get through this and have no choice'. Now I feel I shouldn't clean. I worked in Sainsbury's [a large supermarket chain], but I wasn't a supervisor. After my clinical attachment, I did a day's phlebotomy course and worked as a phlebotomist for a while.
>
> Otmane El Mezoued, refugee doctor from Algeria

> The years out of medicine are a great problem for refugee doctors. Get in touch with good refugee agencies like RETAS to find out about doing PLAB. Do a clinical attachment after PLAB 1 as preparation for PLAB 2. Join refugee doctors' study groups. Link in and put your name on the refugee doctors' database.
>
> Yong Lok Ong, consultant old age psychiatrist from Singapore and
> Overseas Doctors Dean, London Deanery

Fleeing your home and country and starting again as a refugee is never easy. It is estimated that there are between 1500 to 2000 refugee doctors. Most are out of clinical practice, either living off benefits or doing menial, unskilled jobs. Many have spent a decade or more trying to re-establish themselves as practising doctors. This creates an additional problem: time away from medicine makes starting work again difficult. This is compounded when your new country has a different culture.

Help is available. Each deanery has a dean with special responsibility for overseas doctors, who will advise and support refugee doctors. BMA membership is free to refugee doctors, but many are not registered with the GMC, so are not eligible. However, the BMA has a free package – including subscription to the *BMJ*, BMA news, access to the BMA library, and BMA counselling service – and this is available for refugee doctors regardless of whether they are registered with the GMC.

Becoming attached to a network that provides practical help, guidance, friendship and emotional support by others in a similar position can only be a good thing. If you register with the BMA's database of refugee doctors, you will get a free regular newsletter, keeping you up to date with recent developments. It is also well worth finding out from the overseas doctors' dean if there is a study club for refugee doctors.

> You have to fight and be strong. Never give up. Everyone is capable of being someone.
>
> Anonymous refugee surgeon from the Congo

■ Sickness

What happens when you are unwell? You can't work. You have to phone in sick, i.e. explain your situation. Speak to a senior colleague, then ask someone to phone the following:

* your team's secretary
* medical staffing – give an indication of when you will be back and suggest they book a locum
* the people and places that will expect you – wards, outpatients, teaching sessions.

Contact occupational health if you are absent for more than three days or, when you start a new post, if you have a condition making it likely that you will need sick leave.

■ Sick certificates

If you are absent for more than three days, you need a medical certificate stating the nature of your illness. You will need a further medical certificate if you are absent for longer than seven days.

■ Sick pay

The amount of pay you receive while sick depends on how long you have been employed by the NHS. For instance, once you have worked for four months you are entitled to one month's full pay and two months' half pay. During your second year of NHS employment, this increases to two months' full pay and two months' half pay. After six years' NHS service, allowances rise again: six months' full pay and six months' half pay.

■ Home or away?

Some doctors squirm at the suggestion of being treated at their workplace. Receiving treatment away from work can help demarcate boundaries between seemingly disparate doctor and patient roles. For others, familiar surroundings are reassuring. There may be arrangements for doctors to be treated in neighbouring trusts.

◼ When being a doctor and a patient is a help

Many doctors who have been patients believe their experiences make them better doctors. Vulnerability, dependence and the impact of illness on personal relationships cannot be gleaned easily from textbooks or lectures. This may make you more empathic to future patients.

◼ Stress

People who come from abroad always reach a point where they are at their lowest; they have a good cry and then they can pick up and move on. Every foreigner who comes here does that. Having good colleagues helps, as does having a network of friends from home.

Yong Lok Ong, consultant old age psychiatrist from Singapore and
Overseas Doctors Dean, London Deanery

I wasn't prepared for the UK at all. I had no idea what it would be like. I didn't know what MCQ stood for. I didn't know it got dark at four o'clock in December. I was scared to talk to people because I couldn't understand their accents. It was a real nightmare.

Umesh Prabhu, consultant paediatrician from India

Stressed out? It's hardly surprising. PLAB, visa problems, job applications, missing home – it doesn't even have to be something big. Maybe you've lost your wallet, or the train is late again.

At low levels, increases in stress lead to improved performance. Low-level stress is essential for survival as an international doctor, helping you to learn and produce work to high standards. But when peak performance is reached, further stress has catastrophic results. Typically, tiredness is the first sign. Exhaustion and psychiatric problems follow if stress continues unchecked.

◼ Stress prevention

Getting on top of work

Stress causes a surge of noradrenaline in the synaptic cleft, inducing a feeling of elation. It is also why so many of us put off work until the last minute, chasing the 'deadline high'. Its flipside is that when unexpected things happen, like being told your landlord wants to repossess the flat he has been renting to you, or failing an exam, a catastrophic crisis occurs. Stress levels soar.

Set aside time each week for planning and organising work. Sunday evenings can be good for this. Consider using a daily 'to do' list. Ticking things as you do them is strangely addictive and gives you a buzz as you realise how much you've achieved. Everyone puts off things they don't like. Identify high-priority tasks. Do these first and stop them piling up. Don't forget to include enjoyable activities on your list: a meal with friends, a film or football training.

Concentration spans rarely exceed 45 minutes. You need a break after this. Everybody has times when they feel sluggish. Are you an early bird, post-prandial procrastinator or night owl? Identify your least productive time. Use it for flat hunting or updating your CV, not for practising viva technique.

Chunk it up
If you can't eat a big bar of chocolate in one go, you break it up into bits. Why not do the same with work? If an application form is daunting, fill it in stages – a bit every night.

Perfectionism is pointless
Impossibly high self-imposed standards cause stress. Are you working hard, studying, locuming in your spare time to send money home *and* looking after a new baby? Prioritise, and learn to say no.

■ Bad (but common) ways to cope with stress

Alcohol
At first, alcohol makes you feel relaxed. For most doctors, social drinking doesn't become a problem. But if you regularly use alcohol to solve problems, to sleep or to relax, you're heading for trouble.

Practise safe drinking, at most three to four units. If you have a few alcohol-free days each week, dependence is less likely.

Caffeine
Caffeine raises levels of adrenaline and noradrenaline, making feelings of stress worse. A mug of tea contains the same amount of caffeine as a cup of instant coffee.

Smoking
So smoking makes you feel relaxed? Try this. Take your pulse before and after a cigarette. Enough said.

■ Better ways to cope with stress

Exercise
Any sustained regular exercise triggers a chemical reaction in the body, producing hormones called endorphins. These endorphins produce a natural high, which is why you feel good after strenuous physical activity. It doesn't necessarily mean the gym – dancing produces endorphins too.

Relax
Find a way to relax and practise it often. It might be soaking in a candle-lit bath, with your favourite music, followed by a massage. Think back to how you relaxed as a medical student. Just because you are a doctor doesn't mean you have to put away your paintbrushes or flute.

Talking

If you feel stressed, it is likely you are not alone. Find someone to grumble with for half an hour. You will probably feel better. If you are sliding down the slippery stress slope, tell a friend. They can help you find appropriate help and give you the courage to speak to your consultant or tutor before you start to underperform. Making mistakes and failing exams will make you feel worse.

Counselling

Consider paying a visit to occupational health or your GP and ask to be referred to a counsellor. Counsellors are trained to help you find solutions to problems. Your first 'session' will be an assessment. You will usually be seen in a comfortable private room, without interruptions, for about 50 minutes. You will have a chance to describe how you feel. The counsellor will try to understand more about you and how best to help you. Sometimes they suggest other agencies more suited to your needs (*see* Box 7.1). If you both agree counselling could help you, you will be offered a course of 'sessions'. Ten sessions is a typical amount.

Take up a hobby

Squash, chess, flower arranging, pottery – the list is endless.

A friend in need

Maybe your friend is in trouble? You might not know what to say or do. If an international doctor you know is stressed and upset, how should you react?

Do:

* listen and let them know you want to help
* help them find professional advice if you are out of your depth.

Don't:

* tell them what to do. Your best solution might not work for them
* break confidentiality unless you are worried about their safety.

Box 7.1 Helplines and contacts

Local resources
* Your consultant, postgraduate dean or tutor
* GP or occupational health centre
* Hospital chaplaincy (not just for Christians)

National resources
Alcoholics Anonymous
Tel: 07904 644 026
Your first stop for confidential information, help and advice about drinking. Call if you are worried about your drinking, or get advice for your friends.

BMA Counselling Service
Tel: 08459 200 169
A confidential telephone counselling service for BMA members (including medical student members) and their families.

Depression Alliance
35 Westminster Bridge Road
London
SE1 7JB
Tel: 020 7633 9929
Depression Alliance provides information, support and advice for people experiencing depression and their carers.

Eating Disorders Association
1st Floor
103 Prince of Wales Road
London
NR1 1DW
Tel: 01603 621 414 (9am–6.30pm, Mon–Fri)
Website: www.edauk.com
Email: info@edauk.com
Information and advice on eating disorders for sufferers and their friends. They put people in touch with local help.

Manic Depression Fellowship
21 St George's Road
London
SE1 6ES
Tel: 020 7793 2600 9am–5pm, Mon–Thurs; 9am–4pm, Friday
Support, advice and information for people with manic depression (bipolar illness).

National Drugs Helpline
Healthwise Helpline
1st Floor, Cavern Court
8 Matthew Street
Liverpool
L2 6RE
Tel: 0800 77 66 00 (24-hour freephone)
Helpline offering information, counselling and advice about drug misuse. Refers callers to local agencies.

National Schizophrenia Fellowship
28 Castle Street
Kingston-upon-Thames
Surrey
KT1 1SS
Tel: 020 8547 3937 (office); 020 8974 6814 (advice line, 10am–3pm, Mon–Fri)
Website: www.nsf.org.uk
Email: info@nsf.org.uk

NHS Direct
Tel: 0845 4647
Website: www.nhsdirect.nhs.uk
24-hour helpline for any medical problem, staffed by experienced nurses.

■ References

1 Macpherson W (1999) *The Stephen Lawrence Inquiry.* Report of an inquiry by Sir William Macpherson of Cluny. The Stationery Office, London.

2 Esmail A and Everington S (1993) Racial discrimination against doctors from ethnic minorities. *BMJ.* **306**: 691–2.

3 Esmail A and Everington S (1997) Asian doctors are still being discriminated against. *BMJ.* **314**: 1619.

4 Esmail A, Everington S and Doyle H (1998) Racial discrimination in the allocation of distinction awards? Analysis of award holders by type of award, specialty and region. *BMJ.* **316**: 193–5.

5 Esmail A (1994) Complaints may reflect racism. *BMJ.* **308**: 1373–4.

■ Further reading

Stewart E and Nicholas S (2002) Refugee doctors in the United Kingdom. *BMJ.* **325**: S166.

CHAPTER 8

Living in Britain

We have included a chapter on UK living to help you settle in and make the most of life away from the workplace.

■ Money

> Save a lot of money before you come.
> Anand Sharma, SHO in internal medicine from India

UK currency is pounds sterling. It is issued in pounds (£) and pence (p). One pound contains 100 pence. Notes are available in £50, £20, £10 and £5. Coins are available as £2, £1, 50p, 20p, 10p, 5p, 2p and 1p.

We urge you not to carry large amounts of cash. Never leave your money unattended, even in areas that seem secure like staff rooms and changing rooms.

Bank accounts

UK banks may have affiliations with your home bank. Find out before leaving home. This can speed up opening an account when you get to the UK.

The main high-street banks in the UK are

- NatWest
- HSBC
- Lloyds TSB
- Barclays.

Recently, building societies have taken on functions previously performed only by banks. The main building societies are:

- Abbey
- Halifax
- Woolwich
- Bradford and Bingley
- Alliance and Leicester
- Nationwide
- Cheltenham and Gloucester.

To open a bank account, you need to show as much ID as you can, including your passport. Some branches are relaxed, while others take bureaucracy to extremes. You will also need proof of address: utility bills, a rent book or a lease. In addition, banks will need to see bank statements, a letter from your bank at home and a letter from your employer or locum agency.

Take time to compare different banks. Things you will want to ask about are:

- *Current account.* Open a current account to obtain a switch card and cheque book. There is only a very low interest rate on these accounts, but you will be able to access your money quickly and write cheques for things like rent and deposits, and your salary will be paid directly into it.
- *Switch cards.* These look like credit cards but are used to access automatic teller machines (ATMs) and as debit cards in shops. Debit cards take money directly out of your account.
- *Credit cards.* Unlike debit cards, these allow you to defer payment for a month. However, if you cannot pay your monthly bill, you will be charged a high rate of interest. If you pay late, you will also be charged for this. You will probably need to wait until you have a job and proof of income. However, if the bank is affiliated with your home bank, you might be able to get a credit card immediately.
- *Link.* If your credit or debit card has a link symbol it means you can access your money from thousands of ATMs belonging to other banks and building societies, not just the one your account is with.
- *Online banking.* Most banks have free online banking facilities. You can also try digital banks like www.smile.co.uk, www.firstdirect.com or www.egg.com.
- *Charges.* These vary between banks and different types of account, so ask at your branch.

Bank opening hours are usually 9am to 4.30pm. They are very busy at lunch time and if you go during a lunch break, prepare to spend most of it queueing.

Telephone banking is a useful service for busy doctors who find it hard to get to a bank. You will have access to your bank account and to transactions 24 hours a day from a phone. You will still be able to use all of your bank's high-street facilities, but will be able to pay bills and move money between accounts over the phone.

■ Sending money home

You can send money home in two ways:

1 using a bank: expect to pay at least £10. A priority international payment takes a day, but is much more expensive.
2 send a cheque home for your family to pay into your bank account.

■ Getting a National Insurance number

A National Insurance (NI) number is compulsory for the whole UK workforce. All doctors need to have one and will have payments deducted from their salary each month for NI. It pays for pensions and health services. NI numbers are issued through the Department of Social Security (DSS). Getting an NI number can be slow and frustrating.

Phone 0845 915 7006 and tell them your postcode and employment details. This central office will put you in touch with a local office where you will need to make an appointment. You will need:

- your passport
- a letter confirming your employment
- as much ID as you have (at least two items).

In about eight weeks' time you will receive your number by post.

■ Income tax

Anyone working in the UK has to pay between 10% and 40% in direct tax. Everyone has a tax threshold that changes every year. You can currently earn £4615 per annum before being taxed. If you work less than a full tax year, you may be entitled to a refund. For example, if you leave the UK, you can claim a rebate during the year. Forms for rebates can be ordered from the Inland Revenue (0845 070 0040) or from www.inlandrevenue.gov.uk.

Doctors have income tax deducted from pay automatically. This is called Pay As You Earn (PAYE). Monthly deductions from your salary are calculated by the Inland Revenue, based on your annual salary. The tax year starts in April, but it is likely that you will start work on another month. In practice this means your first pay will be a larger sum than for subsequent months.

However, although doctors are on PAYE, many also find themselves in receipt of untaxed income. You must tell the Inland Revenue about any income where no tax has been deducted at source, for example fees for filling out cremation forms, medical reports and police statements.

■ Tax-deductible expenses

Tax-deductible items are things you have paid for on which you can reclaim the money you have paid in tax. These include annual subscription or retention fees of professional bodies approved by the Inland Revenue. In general this means the BMA, GMC and Royal Colleges. If you are unsure we suggest you contact the Inland Revenue for an up-to-date list.

Since 6 April 2002, tax relief for the use of your own vehicle has been based on Inland Revenue predetermined mileage allowance. Their rate depends on the type of vehicle and any qualifying passengers.

It is also possible that you may be overtaxed. There are two forms you need to know about:

- *Form P60* is sent to you at the end of the tax year (5 April). It is proof of the income you have received and the tax you have paid.
- *Form P45* will be given to you when you leave a job. You will need to give it to the payroll at your next place of work to show how much tax you have been paying. If there is a delay between leaving one job and passing your P45 to your new employer's payroll, you will usually be taxed at a higher emergency rate

until it is sorted out. This can take several months so ensure your new pay section has your P45 promptly.

■ Making sense of your payslip

Every month you will get a payslip that provides a comprehensive breakdown of pay and taxes and any other deductions, including NHS pension contributions or bills relating to hospital accommodation, for example telephone charges. Check your payslip each month to make sure you have not been overcharged.

■ Value Added Tax (VAT)

VAT is an indirect tax, levied on petrol, alcoholic drinks, cigarettes and other consumer goods.

■ **The cost of living**

> For the first year you convert everything into rupees.
> Umesh Prabhu, consultant paediatrician from India

The cost of living in the UK varies. As a rule southern England is more expensive than the Midlands, the North, Scotland, Wales and Northern Ireland. Central London is considered the most expensive place in the UK due to the high cost of housing, public transport, parking and entertainment. In rural areas and smaller towns accommodation may be less expensive, but limited public transport may mean that allowances have to be made for a car which can be expensive. In general, you will be able to live more cheaply near small district general hospitals than close to large teaching hospitals.

■ Average prices
- Room in hospital accommodation: £55 per week
- Sharing a rented flat: £60 per week
- Renting a privately owned bedsit: £100 per week
- Bus pass: £40 per month
- Single train fare: £2.00
- Cup of coffee or tea in hospital canteen: £1.00
- Take-away meal for two: £8.00
- Restaurant meal for two (without wine): between £40 and £70
- Bottle of wine in a restaurant: from £12.00
- Bottle of wine in a supermarket: from £3.75
- Pint of beer in a pub: £2.50
- Glass of wine in a pub: £2.00

■ Supermarkets

The large supermarket chains are *Tesco*, *Sainsbury*, *Safeway* and *Asda*. They are sited close to densely populated areas. Supermarkets sell fresh and frozen food, including ready meals that can be heated in a microwave. They also sell toiletries, cleaning materials and alcoholic drinks. Larger ones sell stationery, clothes, CDs and DVDs, and household good such as bedsheets, towels, kettles, microwaves and toasters.

A guide to supermarket prices
- Loaf of bread: 60p
- Pint of milk: 40p
- Box of tea bags: £1.50
- Jar of coffee: £2.00
- Microwave meal: £3.00
- Pre-packed sandwich: £2.50
- Bar of chocolate: 35p

■ International calls

Get an international calling card. You can buy them at newsagents. They work by phoning from your landline and entering a code. I don't know how they make a profit, but they are infinitely cheaper than BT [British Telecom].

Stephanie Young, SpR psychiatrist from New Zealand

■ **Your health**

■ Doctors

Phone NHS Direct on 0845 4647 and tell them your postcode. Ask for a list of GPs in your area and go there to register with one. Consultations are free, but there is a charge for prescriptions. At the time of writing, NHS prescription charges are £6.40 per item. If you anticipate paying for more than five prescriptions in four months or 14 in 12 months, it is cheaper to buy a pre-payment certificate (PPC). A four-month PPC currently costs £33.40 and a 12-month PPC £91.80. You can apply for a PPC using a form available from high-street chemists, or call 0845 850 0030 to buy one over the phone using a credit or debit card.

Seeing your GP
General practitioners are normally seen by appointment. You can make an appointment in person by attending the surgery and arranging a convenient time with the receptionist or by phoning up. It may take time to get through, especially during busy periods, but on the other hand if you take the time to visit the surgery you will probably have to stand and wait while the receptionist is answering the phone.

GPs see emergency cases at the end of surgery or you may be seen instead of someone who fails to turn up. They call to see patients at home where there is, for example, a housebound elderly person or others too acutely ill to travel. There was a time when GPs did all their own out-of-hours home visits: evenings, night-times and at weekends. This has become increasingly less common and now most surgeries use a deputising service. If you require a GP during one of these periods, phone your surgery and you will be directed to the telephone number of this agency.

■ Dentists

Some dentists practise in health centres on a sessional basis, but the majority practise in separate premises. Dentists can be divided into two broad groups: those who provide a service for NHS patients and those who have severed links with the NHS and work privately as independent dentists. But things are not that straightforward. NHS dentists can also take on private work so, for example, some practitioners will still provide you with a filling but only agree to crown one of your teeth privately. Independent dentists charge patients much more than their NHS counterparts. This is because the NHS subsidises dental treatment. If you see an NHS dentist, you still need to pay 75% of the cost of your treatment, but the prices are lower.

Most dentists are listed in the *Yellow Pages*. If you register with an NHS dentist and leave more than 15 months between appointments, you will be removed from their register. NHS Direct will also be able to tell you about local NHS dentists. In some parts of the country many NHS dentists have long waiting lists to join their books.

Emergency dental treatment

Some teaching hospitals have walk-in emergency dental services. Attendance is for a one-off visit to relieve pain. This service is often provided by supervised dental students on a first-come, first-served basis. You may have a long wait. Children and those with severe dental problems are given priority. If you are not sure where the nearest emergency dentist is, either call the dentist you have registered with (there should be a recorded message telling you where to go in an emergency) or look up your nearest one in the *Yellow Pages*. You will be charged standard NHS rates (*see* Box 8.1) for all treatment you receive, whichever emergency clinic you attend.

Box 8.1 NHS dental charges

- Basic examination: from £5.48
- Extensive clinical examination: from £8.20
- Simple scale and polish: from £8.64
- Two small X-rays and one small filling: from £9.60
- One large filling: from £15.08
- A precious metal crown: from £75.64
- A full set of dentures: from £118.88

■ Accommodation

> I have lived in a number of converted flats and think they are quite good, but accommodation here is very expensive. It is not ideal to keep renting alone.
>
> Stephanie Young, SpR psychiatrist from New Zealand

> I hardly know my neighbours. I know one of them has a dog because I hear the dog barking.
>
> Anuga Shedeo, PLAB candidate from India

Some doctors arriving in the UK might be lucky enough to have family or friends that they can stay with until they have found their feet. Others will not. This section provides an overview of the UK housing sector to help you find your way around.

■ Where to find accommodation

There are various ways of finding somewhere to live. Flats, flat-shares and rooms for rent are advertised through a range of media. Local newspapers, hospital newsletters and student magazines carry classified advertisements. Many small corner shops display adverts for accommodation alongside those from childminders, plumbers, retired gentlemen prepared to work on your garden or someone needing to sell their prized collection of Elvis records. Landlords and people looking for someone to share a flat put handwritten or typed adverts on doctors' mess or staff canteen notice boards and others just ask accommodation managers if they know of somebody who is looking. Estate agents offer rental properties as well as houses and flats for sale and others act as agents to help you find a place to rent.

■ Accommodation options

- Staying with family or friends. If you have family or friends prepared to put you up, you have a head start. Rent and other housing costs are expensive. Landlords expect money upfront, e.g. rent in advance, a deposit (returnable when you move out) and other fees such as reconnection to a telephone line.
- Hostels are a makeshift solution. Generally they consist of a basic room that may be shared and shared access to a shower and toilet. Cooking facilities are limited or non-existent so eating out may become an expensive necessity.
- Single or married hospital accommodation is cheaper than comparable privately rented accommodation. Married accommodation is much harder to get hold of. The hospital will have an accommodation officer who should be able to help. Contact her early. She will probably have lists of local landlords if the hospital is unable to provide you with the sort of accommodation you need, for example if you have a family.
- A hospital-owned rented flat or part of a house has much going for it. It will usually be near your workplace, ruling out an immediate need for a car or costly bus or train journeys. These places are generally furnished so you will

not have to buy plates, cooking equipment, a fridge, bedding and somewhere to keep your clothes. Bathrooms and kitchens may be shared. This can be a mixed blessing in that you might have the opportunity to make friends with others in the kitchen and share chores and ingredients. The disadvantage of living near or in your hospital is that you can get trapped. It could be difficult to get away from your place of work, especially if town is some distance away.

- Renting a privately owned flat or house will depend on a number of factors, including what the property is like and its suitability for your needs, e.g. its nearness to shops and your workplace, schools for your children and whether the area is secure. To be truly happy you need a trusting relationship with your landlord. We advise you to sign provided formal contracts that spell out the terms of your agreement.
- Buying your own property is a huge commitment. Most international doctors feel they have enough to organise, without the additional worry of estate agents, mortgages, insurance, security and needing to sell a house when they return home.

Almost all SHO and SpR rotations include jobs in different hospitals. These may be considerable distances from each other and from your accommodation.

Whichever form of accommodation you get, all the following agencies need to be informed when you move in.

■ Council

Council tax pays for local services, including libraries, refuse collection and the police. The local council will tell you how much it is. You can pay in monthly instalments.

■ Television licence

You need to have a television licence if you have a television. You need one for your television even if you live in communal accommodation where other residents have licences for their televisions.

■ Utility providers: gas, electricity, water, sewerage and telephone

Bills are not included for most rented accommodation. It is important to have baseline electricity and gas meter readings taken when you move in so that you don't end up paying for the previous occupants.

■ Contents insurance

This covers personal possessions in your accommodation, for example your clothes, stereo system and books. Look in the *Yellow Pages* for insurance companies or ask the accommodation officer. It is worth phoning several as quotes vary.

■ Transport

> When I first came here I used to take public transport: the underground
> and bus. Nobody talked. Everybody was there but they didn't speak.
>
> Otmane El Mezoued, refugee doctor from Algeria

■ Trains

> What confused me was the difference in ticket price. I was shocked. In the
> early morning, to go from Manchester to London costs £117. When you
> realise that if you book in advance it is only £25, you just feel like banging
> your head against a wall. Nobody tells you this information; you find out
> by chance.
>
> Umesh Prabhu, consultant paediatrician from India

British railways can be confusing. Vastly different prices for the same journey
seem baffling. To get a better understanding of what has been called British
Railways, British Rail or the Rail Network, it is worth going back to how it all
started.

Steam locomotives were invented in England. The earliest railway lines were
constructed here and an industry started. The technology and expertise were
exported all over the globe and it could be argued that every other railway has
benefited from mistakes made here. Unlike most European cities which have one
large central railway station, London and a number of other British cities and
towns have more than one large railway station. This is because early railways
and trains were built by private firms and often more than one company were
competing for a similar route.

London has a number of major railway stations and so it is possible, for
example, to travel to the West Country from Paddington or Waterloo, and to the
North of England and Scotland from Euston or King's Cross.

The private companies running the different routes were taken over by the state
in the late 1940s after the Second World War. During the Conservative Thatcher and
Major years (1979–1997), the railway structure was broken up with one company
looking after the railway lines and other companies providing and operating
trains. Poor service, like the weather, is a topic of conversation between strangers
waiting for an overdue train. It produces hours of agreeable huffing and puffing.
Indeed, many English people almost seem to enjoy grumbling about poor punctuality,
delays, lack of information from staff, vandalism to stations and carriages, graffiti
and unhygienic toilets!

First-class ticket holders pay a lot more for very little extra, and the cost of
the same journey varies enormously depending on whether you buy the ticket
in advance, travel after the morning rush hour or at the weekend. Students and
pensioners can buy a card that entitles them to big discounts, but there are
restrictions on when they can travel. For example, discounts might not be available on bank holidays. Don't expect much help from station staff. Information
desks are often unstaffed, and when staff are there you can expect a long wait
behind a queue of people with a series of complex and unrelated questions. It is
better to do your own research online.

Despite these shortcomings, the UK has a comprehensive railway system and it is an ideal way of getting a feel for cities, towns and countryside. You are afforded views of private back gardens, often more interesting than formal fronts. The countryside is frequently stunning and varied and there is no better way of seeing it than through a train window.

In addition to the nationwide rail network, there are local networks servicing major cities. London, while known for its underground (the tube), is also served by many small stations.

Qjump and The Trainline
Qjump and The Trainline are online services where you can search by fastest journey or cheapest ticket, store favourite journeys and buy securely online.

PlusBus
PlusBus is a combined train and bus ticket that gives you unlimited travel on most buses at either one or both ends of a rail journey. PlusBus tickets can be bought as add-ons to any rail journey that starts or finishes at participating stations, and give you access to the bus network in that area for 24 hours. Since October 2002, 135 stations have incorporated the PlusBus scheme, and it will be progressively rolled out across the country.

Buses and coaches
Bus or coach travel falls into three groups:

- long-distance coaches
- local buses
- excursion buses for local hire.

Long-distance coaches
Long-distance coaches are a cheaper alternative to trains. A huge network fans out of Victoria Coach Station in London. Victoria Coach Station opened in 1932. With only a brief and enforced interruption during part of the Second World War, the company provided London terminal facilities for its shareholding operators and their passengers through the pre-war growth and postwar decline of the industry. In 1988, Victoria Coach Station was bought by London Transport.

Most long-distance coaches are comfortable and have a toilet. By using motorways, they cover large distances almost as fast as trains.

Local buses
Every city or town has a bus service that is used to take workers and others to and from the centre. Standards vary. The top floor of a double-decker bus gives passengers a great view, especially from the front seats. There are also rural bus services used by local commuters and schoolchildren, but these run less frequently.

Excursion buses for local hire
The UK has hundreds of private bus companies. They provide, for example, school runs and excursions. Some go across the Channel to France and beyond. They are popular with the elderly but also useful to families who don't have a car but perhaps want to visit the seaside or other places of interest.

■ Taxis

Expect to pay more on bank holidays, at night-time and for telephone bookings.

■ Cars

> In India somebody puts petrol in your car, and so the first time I went to
> the petrol station I was waiting for somebody to come and put petrol in.
>   Umesh Prabhu, consultant paediatrician from India

Cars are useful if you have small children or anticipate making frequent trips around the UK. Buying a new car is expensive. Second-hand cars can be bought from second-hand car dealers. They are also advertised in local newspapers, hospital newsletters, in a magazine called *Autotrader*, and you will see signs on cars on the road indicating that they are for sale. Both the Automobile Association (AA) and Royal Automobile Club (RAC) will inspect a second-hand car and advise you. It costs around £100. You can drive in the UK for a year on the driving licence from your own country. You will then either be able to swap it for a British licence or you may need to take a driving test (*see* Box 8.2).

Box 8.2 Driving Licence Regulations	
European Economic Area	A full driving licence issued in any EEA country can be swapped for a British licence.
Gibraltar	A full driving licence issued in Gibraltar can be swapped for a British licence.
Australia Austria Barbados British Virgin Islands Cyprus Finland Hong Kong Japan Kenya Malta New Zealand Singapore Sweden Switzerland Zimbabwe	A full driving licence issued in any of these countries can be swapped for a British licence.

| Any other country | A driving licence from any other country cannot be swapped for a British licence. After using your licence for a year, you will have to take a driving test. If you are unsuccessful you can drive on a provisional licence, but someone with a full driving licence must accompany you at all times and the car must display a red L plate, indicating you are a learner driver. |

You will need to buy a tax disc and display it on your front windscreen if you are keeping or using a vehicle on the road. The disc can be bought at the Post Office. You will need to show an insurance certificate and MOT certificate.

Insurance
It is illegal to drive a car without insurance. There are three types:

- *third party* – if you have an accident, this pays for damage to the other car only
- *third part, fire and theft* – this pays for damage to another vehicle if you have an accident, but also covers your car against fire damage and theft
- *comprehensive* – this covers you for damage to your own car, and fire and theft. You will usually have to pay an excess charge, typically the first £100 of any claim.

Shop around for insurance. A few hours spent phoning a number of companies (advertised in the *Yellow Pages*) and getting a competitive quote is well spent. Bigger, faster cars are more expensive to insure. Several other factors affect your premium: your age, keeping the car in a secure garage, anit-theft devices and the area you live in are all taken into account.

MOT certificate
If your car is more than three years old, you have to take it for a yearly Ministry of Transport (MOT) test. MOTs take about 20 minutes. A registered car mechanic goes through a comprehensive checklist that covers everything to do with car safety. Steering, brakes, lights and tyres are all tested. MOT tests are done at testing centres and local garages. The test costs around £30. If a car fails the test, it must undergo relevant repairs and be retested. It is illegal to drive a car without a valid MOT.

Parking
Parking can be problematic. Many hospitals operate a 'pay and display' system. To park at others you may need a permit, which can cost up to £200 a year. There is a waiting list for permits in many larger hospitals and preference is often given to permanent staff.

■ Transport contact details

UK Public Transport Information: www.pti.org.uk
National Rail: www.nationalrail.co.uk/
PlusBus: www.plusbus.info/index.htm
Qjump: www.qjump.co.uk
The Trainline: www.thetrainline.com
National Express (coaches): www.nationalexpress.com
Driving and Vehicle Licensing Agency (DVLA): 0870 240 0009

■ Child care

> Don't take risks. If in doubt get your kid out.
> Ashraf Khan, staff grade paediatrician from Pakistan

By law, children aged between five and 16 have to attend school. State schools are free. Private schools are expensive and beyond what most junior doctors can afford. Many children under five go to nursery school. Again there are both state-run and private nursery schools, but state nurseries get full quickly, so you may have to pay. It is against the law to leave children under 14 unattended by a responsible adult.

Unless you are fortunate enough to have a family member who is prepared to look after your young children, you can anticipate paying considerable sums to have them looked after while you are at work (*see* Box 8.3).

Box 8.3 Child-care options

- A live-in nanny
- A nanny who comes to your house while you are working
- A live-in au pair
- A place in a hospital crèche
- A local authority or private nursery
- A registered child-minder

■ Nannies

Nannies have a recognised qualification and/or are very experienced in child care. A nanny is supposed to stimulate your children's physical, intellectual and social development. They also carry out nursery duties, including preparing children's meals, laundry, school runs and tidying the child's bedroom. Their salary depends on their age, experience and qualification, and also on whether they are required to live in with the family or live out. They are expensive to employ (£8–£10 per hour); realistically, the only people who can afford to use a nanny are couples where both partners are earning consultant salaries. Everyone else looks for a less expensive option.

■ Au pair

The au pair scheme allows unmarried people (usually women), aged between 17 and 27, with no dependants to come to the UK to learn English. An au pair lives with an English-speaking family as part of the household. In return for helping about the home and with child care for a maximum of five hours per day, the au pair receives 'pocket money', around £50 per week, and has at least two free days per week.

Whether this arrangement works depends on the personality and aptitude of the au pair, the relationship they are able to form with your child or children, and their maturity. It also depends on how well they are managed by you and on what has motivated them to come to the UK.

■ Hospital crèche or nursery

These look after pre-school-age children. You can expect to pay around £1.80 per child per hour. Where a hospital crèche or nursery is available, there is often a shortage of places. Some only offer places during office hours so may be of limited use. Often fines are imposed if you are late arriving to collect your child, even if this is due to a clinical emergency. Another difficulty is that the care on offer is institutional with different nursery nurses looking after your child from day to day.

■ Local authority or private nurseries

While it is usually cheaper and more convenient to have your pre-school-age child cared for at your hospital, this may not be possible. Most full-time nurseries are open 8am–6pm, five days a week. But with any nursery, you may find it is difficult to get in as demand outweighs the number of available places. Some private nurseries receive state subsidy and they can be the least expensive form of child care. Find the locations of as many state and private nurseries as you can and keep in mind the following criteria:

1 What are the staff and facilities like? Staff may be nursery nurses, teachers, nurses, playleaders or unqualified. Check the ratio of staff to children.
2 Do you feel safe leaving your child with them?
3 What sort of stimulation and activities are offered?
4 What procedures are in place for emergencies?
5 How near is it to my home or workplace?
6 How easy is it to get there during the school run and other busy times?
7 How sympathetic are staff to a child's needs? Will they provide vegetarian meals, for instance?
8 What do other parents think?
9 What contingencies could be put in place in the event of my being delayed at work?
10 Always trust your instincts: if in doubt go elsewhere.

■ Registered child-minders

Child-minders are usually experienced mothers who have elected to stay at home to look after their own children and take in a small number of other people's children to earn extra money. They care for children up to the age of eight years in their own home. Anyone who cares for children for more than two hours in a day, for pay or other reward, is required under the Children Act 1989 to register with their local social services department as a child-minder. Most registered child-minders provide full day care for children during the week.

Local authorities have child-minder coordinators who are employed to provide contact details and also ensure that children are being looked after responsibly. Our experience suggests they assess tangible factors such as the physical environment, but not factors such as how good someone is with other people's children.

Therefore you will need to address all the same questions as for nurseries. Check out the childminder's house for clues:

- Are the other children enjoying themselves?
- Are pets under control?
- Do the toys, books and minder show a positive attitude to children of your cultural background?
- Is there somewhere quiet for children to rest?

Observe how they treat their own children. Make a second visit to the ones you like most and ask if you can contact another parent as a referee. Make sure you see the child-minder's current registration certificate and confirmation of annual inspection.

Child-minder rates depend on hours and meals and range from £2.50 to £5 per child per hour. Ensure that you make a good written contract with your child-minder and provide details of how you can be contacted in an emergency. Make sure that you pay at agreed intervals. Like the best grandmothers or aunts, the best child-minders are worth their weight in gold. Make sure they feel valued.

Doctors, unlike nurseries and child-minders, work unsocial hours. This can make child care a challenge, particularly for school-age children. You may need to combine one or more options. Some doctors pair up and arrange to have each other's children when the other is on call.

■ Child-care contacts

National Child-minding Association
8 Masons Hill
Bromley
Kent
BR2 9EY
Tel: 020 8464 6164
Fax: 020 8290 6834
Website: www.ncma.org.uk

Daycare Trust is the national child-care campaign and advises parents. Tel: 020 7840 3350 (10am–5pm, Mon–Fri)
Website: www.daycaretrust.org.uk

■ Entertainment

> When I first came to England I was based in Devon. Later I moved to London and it was a culture shock. I liked the vibe and knew that this was the place I wanted to hang out in for a few years.
>
> Stephanie Young, SpR psychiatrist from New Zealand

> Everyone is different: one person might like to go to the gym, another might play golf, but every human being needs something different to do. You can see things more clearly when you are a few steps away. It's healthy and useful to have very different interests.
>
> Zerrin Atakan from Turkey, Lead Consultant, National Psychosis Unit

In a book like this we can't do justice to this topic. We provide merely a short introduction and a few suggestions. As visitors to London who buy a copy of *Time Out* will testify, every morning, afternoon, evening and night can be enjoyably passed one hundred times over. This may not be the case in Chipping Sodbury, Pratt's Bottom or Ilkley Moor, but generally if you are tired of Britain you are tired of life.

Apart from magazines like *Time Out* and *What's On*, Londoners also have the *Evening Standard* and national broadsheets to tell them what they can expect for entertainment. There are always things going on in the Royal Albert Hall, Royal Festival Hall, Barbican and numerous other venues. Other cities have local news-papers and magazines where entertainments are advertised.

> In hospital you are cosseted by colleagues, but you need a life outside of hospital too. British people are not too good at socialising outside.
>
> Yong Lok Ong, consultant old age psychiatrist from Singapore
> and Overseas Doctors Dean, London Deanery

■ Sport

London is home to Chelsea, Arsenal, Fulham, Charlton Athletic and Tottenham Hotspur football clubs; in total there are 13 professional football clubs in Greater London. Be warned, the popularity of the Premiership means that top fixtures are sold out well in advance. However, if you are just interested in sampling a game you shouldn't have difficulty watching lower division sides like Brentford, Queen's Park Rangers or Leyton Orient. This applies to lower division sides across the country.

Cricket fans know that England houses Lords, The Oval, Trent Bridge and Old Trafford. Once again, getting tickets for test matches may be difficult but county fixtures shouldn't cause you any problems.

Other sports like rugby, hockey (land and ice), athletics, tennis and swimming are all catered for in the capital and elsewhere.

■ Music

Every musical taste is catered for, especially in London and other large centres. If you like classical music there are professional resident orchestras based in Birmingham, Manchester, Liverpool and Bournemouth. London has many orchestras. Concerts take place most days somewhere in the capital between September and June. There are numerous chamber groups to be found. Opera is catered for at Covent Garden and the Coliseum in London. Both companies tour throughout the UK. If you play an orchestral instrument to a reasonable standard, there are many amateur orchestras that will happily give you an audition.

If you prefer jazz, the world-famous Ronnie Scott's Club can be found in Frith Street in London where there is jazz seven nights a week. There is a Ronnie Scott's Club in Birmingham as well and many other jazz venues throughout the UK.

All the world's touring rock bands perform in London in venues such as Earl's Court or Wembley Arena. They also perform at other major centres, e.g. the National Exhibition Centre (NEC) in Birmingham and the Milton Keynes Bowl.

■ Art

Every large town and city has its civic art gallery, usually housing a permanent collection that is supplemented by travelling or ad hoc exhibitions. Once again Londoners are spoilt for choice with the National, National Portrait Gallery, Tate, Tate Britain and other important collections. Many of these galleries have no admission fee (although you will be asked for a donation). The Royal Academy Summer Exhibition in Burlington House is always worth a visit as it contains a vast array of art in numerous styles. Anyone can submit their work for selection and it is judged by the hanging committee. The Victoria and Albert Museum houses a huge collection of artefacts, fabrics, pottery, metalwork and sculpture and is also worth visiting.

■ From Hollywood to Bollywood

Cinemas are everywhere. Old town centre cinemas are slowly being replaced by multiplexes, located either in new shopping centres or outside towns on trading estates. Despite many screens, the choice of film is often restricted to Hollywood blockbusters and other commercial films. It is unlikely that you will be able to find art house or foreign (non-English) films in these complexes. There are some independent cinemas run by enthusiasts for film buffs, but outside big cities these are few and far between. London houses the National Film Theatre. This is a remarkable establishment which, in addition to film seasons where you can follow the work of, say, Cary Grant, Alfred Hitchcock or Richard Attenborough, puts on special events such as live interviews with, for example, Woody Allen.

■ Comedy

Comedy is the new rock and roll. Comedy clubs have sprung up like mushrooms in recent years, many disappearing almost as quickly. Standards vary, but it is likely that this period will be remembered as a golden era in decades to come as there are now so many varied and talented performers. Most comedy has moved away from traditional mother-in-law jokes to powerful observational comedy with a left of centre political slant. Performers often pick on members of the audience, so we advise you not to sit near the front.

■ Dance

Ballet dancing can be seen at Sadler's Wells Theatre and Covent Garden where there are resident companies. These and others tour the provinces. Ballroom dancing may not quite have the hold it once had on middle England, but there is still a string of ballroom dancing schools dotted around the UK where you can learn to waltz, brush up your tango and quicken your quickstep.

■ Clubbing

London is the centre of the world clubbing scene. Clubbing has a distinct culture and rules. Since the late 1980s UK nightclubs have revolutionised global dance music. Clubbing is not new, but has moved up from underground and become more accessible. Nightclub entry will cost between £10 and £15. There are often special deals and discounts if you have a flyer or arrive early.

To have a fantastic experience, you need to follow a few rules. Expect to be searched for drugs when entering a club. Bouncers are often verbally aggressive. Don't try to talk your way in or jump the queue. Don't be rude or overfamiliar with them. Carry enough cash to get home safely. Taxis cost more at night and in the early hours of the morning. Night buses can be unsafe and there will probably not be any other forms of public transport. Take change for the cloakroom. They charge around £1–£2 per item, so don't take a full change of clothes. Don't leave your drinks unattended as someone might tamper with them.

■ Drinking

Colleagues may suggest 'going for a drink' after work. Unwinding and chatting over a drink in a public house (pub) is a good way to get to know your new colleagues. You don't have to order an alcoholic drink and many pubs serve food. This tends to be cheaper than eating out in a restaurant.

Consuming alcoholic beverages in the company of others is perhaps Britain's second favourite pastime, after television. International doctors can practise their skill in what is euphemistically called 'elbow lifting' in hospital social clubs before graduating to pubs. These vary enormously from quaint country inns (the sort you see on Christmas cards) with a crackling log fire, horse brass ornaments and traditional pub food at one end of the spectrum through to pubs of the 'spit and sawdust' variety. These latter establishments will be familiar to readers of Hardy and Dickens. It should be noted that beer is usually bought as draught, from a barrel. It is ordered in pints or half pints. A pint is a little over half a litre. Spirits (sometimes known as shorts) like whisky, gin, vodka and rum are measured in gills. House wine can be bought by the glass, in a small or large measure. Pub measures of wine vary from 50–250 ml. Non-alcoholic alternatives like fruit juice or cola are always available and it is often possible to get tea or coffee. It could be argued that teetotal customers can have just as enjoyable a time as their alcohol-consuming companions and may even remember more about their time in the pub the following day.

The UK has stringent drink–driving laws and the police are able to breathalyse any motorist they think may have consumed alcohol. It is imperative that you do not drink and drive as the penalties are severe and could have an adverse effect on your career.

■ Public libraries

A number of international doctors have told us how much they value public libraries. Large towns and cities have big central libraries and they are readily available and free to members of the public. The older ones were often funded by local phil-anthropists, while newer ones tend to be built by local authorities. Provided you have proof of local residence you can easily get a library ticket. A utility bill from British Telecom, a council tax demand or a rent book with your name and address will do. This card not only allows you to borrow books from your local branch, but others connected to it electronically. So, for example, if you join the Dartford branch in Kent, you can borrow books elsewhere in the county, and if you join the Bexleyheath central library your ticket lets you borrow from other libraries in Greater London.

Many small towns and even villages have a library, but of necessity the stock may be limited and the opening hours restricted. Some rural areas are even provided with a mobile library van, bringing books to people who may have difficulty getting to town.

Public libraries have large collections of fiction and non-fiction books across an array of subjects. Many libraries have branched out into other media and it is possible to borrow music CDs, videos and even paintings. Some have exhibition space used for art, photography or mixed media shows, either of local talent or touring national exhibits. Most have children's sections, as there is an ethos of bringing on the next generation of readers. Children's librarians sometimes lay on special events such as readings by authors or performances by storytellers.

The number of books that you can borrow varies, but couples or families with more than one ticket will be able to take out more than they need. Your book is stamped with a 'return by' date and if you fail to bring it in by then you are expected to pay a fine, which progressively increases as weeks and months tick by. However, a book may be renewed over the phone unless someone else has ordered it.

You too can order books if the one you are looking for is not in stock. Enquiry desks have pre-printed postcards – all you have to do is fill in your address and book details, pay a nominal administrative charge and wait.

■ Reference libraries

Larger town and city libraries usually have a reference library attached to their borrowing section. It contains reference books, magazines, newspapers and other useful material that can be read on the premises but not removed. Many now have computers providing internet access where you can book slots and most have facilities for scanning old land records and other documents on microfilm. These establishments have collections of telephone directories and *Yellow Pages* (which carries information about businesses listed by trade) for the whole country, not just the local area. Your household will only be supplied with a telephone directory and *Yellow Pages* for your local area, so this is a useful way of obtaining contact details for a person or business in another region.

Reference reading rooms are places where you can find all human life, from tramps escaping to a place of comparative comfort and warmth, to schoolchildren diligently working on a project, to an autodidact hunting for a historical nugget hidden away on microfilm.

Librarians are remarkably helpful. There are two types: trained librarians and library assistants who stamp books and carry out the bulk of mundane duties. Trained librarians are often extremely knowledgeable and will be able to find reference sources for you very quickly.

Libraries are also a useful source of local information. Many have lists of clubs, societies and organisations in their locality. The details of each are kept on a computer file and can be accessed by members of the public. Most are keen for new members. They also provide information on evening classes run by local authorities – another easy way to pick up new skills and make friends.

■ Evening classes and adult education

> Joining associations you are interested in helps you develop a sense of belonging. I joined the oriental ceramic society where I met people with the same interest. I encourage people to join societies or play sport with indigenous people.
>
> Yong Lok Ong, consultant old age psychiatrist from Singapore and
> Overseas Doctors Dean, London Deanery

These are administered by local authorities. Courses are inexpensive and sometimes free, but the subjects you can study vary. Small centres may be restricted to old favourites like pottery, flower arranging, cookery and computer skills, while in large cities just about anything can be studied. In London, *Floodlight* (available in most larger London newsagents) provides a brief outline of thousands of courses with their costs and contact details. An evening class is a great way to meet other people, and engaging in an actual activity can be much less intimidating than gatherings in a pub.

■ Further reading

1 Mikes G (1970) *How to be an Alien*. Penguin, Harmondsworth.

2 Paxman J (1999) *The English: portrait of a people*. Penguin, Harmondsworth.

Common medical/healthcare abbreviations used in Britain

A&E	accident and emergency department
ABG	arterial blood gases
ACE	angiotensin converting enzyme
ACLS	advanced certificate in life support
ACTH	adrenocorticotrophic hormone
ADH	antidiuretic hormone
AF	atrial fibrillation
AHA	area health authorities
AIDS	acquired immune deficiency syndrome
ALL	acute lymphoblastic leukaemia
ALT	alanine transaminase
AML	acute myeloid leukaemia
ANF	antinuclear factor
ARDS	adult respiratory distress syndrome
ASD	atrial septal defect
ASO	antistrepsolysin-O
AST	aspartate transaminase
ATM	automatic teller machine
AXR	abdominal chest X-ray
BBB	bundle branch block
BIBA	brought in by ambulance
BMA	British Medical Association
CABG	coronary artery bypass graft
CAH	chronic active hepatitis
CAPD	chronic ambulatory peritoneal dialysis
CCF	congestive cardiac failure
CCST	Certificate of Completion of Specialist Training
CCU	coronary care unit
CD	controlled drugs
CHI	Commission for Health Improvement (now the Healthcare Commission)
CLL	chronic lymphatic leukaemia
CML	chronic myeloid leukaemia
CMV	cytomegalovirus
CNS	central nervous system
CPD	continuing professional development
CPN	community psychiatric nurses
CPR	cardiopulmonary resuscitation
CRF	chronic renal failure; corticotrophin releasing factor
CSF	cerebrospinal fluid
CSM	Committee for Safety in Medicines
CT	computerised tomography

CVA	cerebrovascular accident
CVP	central venous pressure
CVS	cardiovascular system
CXR	chest X-ray
DCH	Diploma of Child Health
DIC	disseminated intravascular coagulopathy
DNA	did not attend
DOA	dead on arrival
DoH	Department of Health
DSS	Department of Social Security
DU	duodenal ulcer
DVT	deep venous thrombosis
Dx or Δ	diagnosis
EBV	Epstein–Barr virus
ECG	electrocardiograph
ECJ	European Court of Justice
EEA	European Economic Area
EEG	electroencephalograph
EMQ	extended matching question
EMU	early morning urine
ENT	ear, nose and throat
ERCP	endoscopic retrograde cholangiopancreatography
ESR	erythrocyte sedimentation rate
EWTD	European Working Time Directive
FBC	full blood count
FFP	fresh frozen plasma
FRCA	Fellow of the Royal College of Anaesthetists
FTN	fixed-term training number
FTTA	fixed term training appointment
GMC	General Medical Council
GMS	general medical services
GP	general practitioner
GPwSI	general practitioner(s) with a special interest
HLA	human leucocyte antigen
HOCM	hypertrophic obstructive cardiomyopathy
HPC	history of presenting complaint
HR	human resources
ICU	intensive care unit
ID	identification
IELTS	International English Language Testing System
IHD	ischaemic heart disease
IM	intramuscular
INR	international normalised ratio
IT	information technology
ITU	intensive therapy unit
IVU	intravenous urography
JCPTGP	Joint Committee on Postgraduate Training for General Practice
JVP	jugular venous pressure
LAD	left axis deviation

LAS	locum appointment for service
LAT	locum appointment for training
LBBB	left bundle-branch block
LDA	Locum Doctors Association
LDL	low-density lipoprotein
LFT	liver function test
LH	luteinising hormone
LVF	left ventricular failure
MCQ	multiple-choice question
MCV	mean corpuscular volume
MFPH	Member of the Faculty of Public Health
MI	myocardial infarction
MRCGP	Member of the Royal College of General Practitioners
MRCOG	Member of the Royal College of Obstetricians and Gynaecologists
MRCP	Member of the Royal College of Physicians
MRCPath	Member of the Royal College of Pathologists
MRCPCH	Member of the Royal College of Paediatrics and Child Health
MRCPsych	Member of the Royal College of Psychiatrists
MRCS	Member of the Royal College of Surgeons
MRI	magnetic resonance imaging
MSU	mid-stream urine
NBM	nil by mouth
NHS	National Health Service
NICE	National Institute for Clinical Excellence
NTN	national training number
OCP	oral contraceptive pill
ODTS	Overseas Doctors Training Scheme
OSCE	objective structured clinical examination
OSPE	objective structured pathology examination
OTC	over the counter
PACES	Practical Assessment of Clinical Examination Skills
PC	presenting complaint
PCP	pneumocystis carinii pneumonia
PCT	primary care trust
PCV	packed cell volume
PDA	patent ductus arteriosus
PEEP	positive end-expiratory pressure
PEFR	peek expiratory flow rate
PET	positron emission tomography
PLAB	Professional and Linguistic Assessments Board
PMP	patient management problem
PMS	personal medical services
POM	prescription-only medicines
PPC	pre-payment certificate
PR	per rectum
PRHO	pre-registration house officer
PRV	polycythaemia rubra vera
PT	prothrombin time
PTH	parathyroid hormone

PTT	partial thromboplastin time
PTTK	partial thromboplastin time with kaolin
PUO	pyrexia of unknown origin
PV	per vagina
Px	prescription
RAD	right axis deviation
RBBB	right bundle-branch block
RCC	red cell concentrate
RF	rheumatoid factor
RHA	regional health authority
RIF	right iliac fossa
RMO	resident medical officer
RUQ	right upper quadrant
RVF	right ventricular failure
Rx	treatment
SACD	subacute combined degeneration
SAS	staff-grade and associate specialists
SBE	subactute bacterial endocarditis
SHO	senior house officer
SLE	systemic lupus erythmatosis
SPECT	single photon emission computerised tomography
SpR	specialist registrar
SVT	supraventricular tachycardia
TIA	transient ischaemic attack
TPN	total parenteral nutrition
TURP	transurethral resection of the prostate
U&E	urea and electrolytes
UK	United Kingdom
URTI	upper respiratory tract infection
USS	ultrasound scan
UTI	urinary tract infection
VDRL	Veneral Diseases Research Laboratory
VF	ventricular fibrillation
VLDL	very low density lipoprotein
VSD	ventricular septal defect
VT	ventricular tachycardia
VTN	visiting training number
VTS	vocational training scheme
VWF	Von Willebrand factor
WBC	white blood cell

Contact information

British Medical Association (BMA)
BMA House
Tavistock Square
London
WC1H 9JR
Tel: 020 7383 6033
Email: info.web@bma.org.uk
Website: www.bma.org.uk
International Department, including Refugees Doctors' Liaison Group:
www.bma.org.uk/international

Faculty of Public Health Medicine
Royal College of Physicians
4 St Andrew's Place
London
NW1 4LB
Tel: 020 7935 0243

Gay and Lesbian Association of Doctors and Dentists (GLADD)
PO Box 5606
London
W4 1WY
Tel: 0870 765 5606
Website: www.gladd.org.uk

General Medical Council (GMC)
178 Great Portland Street
London
W1W 5JE
Tel: 020 7580 7642
Website: www.gmc-uk.org

Royal College of Anaesthetists
48–49 Russell Square
London
WC1B 4JY
Tel: 020 7813 1900
Website: www.rcoa.ac.uk

Royal College of General Practitioners
14 Prince's Gate
London
SW7 1PU
Tel: 020 7581 3232
Website: www.rcgp.org.uk

Royal College of Obstetricians and Gynaecologists
27 Sussex Place
Regent's Park
London
NW1 4RG
Tel: 020 7772 6200
Websites: www.repromed.net and www.rcog.org.uk

Royal College of Ophthalmologists
17 Cornwell Terrace
London
NW1 4QW
Tel: 020 7935 0702
Website: www.rcophth.ac.uk

Royal College of Paediatrics and Child Health
50 Hallum Street
London
WC1N 6DE
Tel: 020 7307 5600
Website: www.rcph.ac.uk

Royal College of Pathologists
2 Carlton House Terrace
London
SW1Y 5AF
Tel: 020 7930 5861
Website: www.rcpath.org

Royal College of Physicians
11 St Andrew's Place
Regent's Park
London
NW1 4LE
Tel: 020 7935 1174
Website: www.rcplondon.ac.uk

Royal College of Physicians and Surgeons of Glasgow
232–42 St Vincent's Street
Glasgow
G2 5RJ
Tel: 0141 221 6072
Website: www.rcpsglasg.ac.uk

Royal College of Physicians of Edinburgh
9 Queen Street
Edinburgh EH2 1JQ
Tel: 0131 225 7324
Website: www.rcpe.ac.uk

Royal College of Physicians of Ireland
6 Kildare Street
Dublin
D2
Tel: 00 353 1 661 6677
Website: www.rcpi.ie/

Royal College of Psychiatrists
17 Belgrave Square
London
SW1X 8PG
Tel: 020 7235 2351
Website: www.rcpsych.ac.uk

Royal College of Radiologists
38 Portland Place
London
W1N 4JQ
Tel: 020 7636 4432
Website: www.rcr.ac.uk

Royal College of Surgeons of Edinburgh
Nicolson Street
Edinburgh
EH8 9DW
Tel: 0131 527 3474
Website: www.rcsed.ac.uk

Royal College of Surgeons of England
35–43 Lincoln's Inn Fields
London
WC2A 3PN
Tel: 020 7405 3474
Website: www.rcseng.ac.uk

Royal College of Surgeons of Ireland
St Stephen's Green
Dublin
D2
Tel: 00 353 1 412 2100
Website: www.rcsi.ie/

Index